Liliane de Fátima F. Gallinea

Swallowing sounds in cerebral palsy using Doppler sonar

Liliane de Fátima F. Gallinea

Swallowing sounds in cerebral palsy using Doppler sonar

ScienciaScripts

Imprint

Any brand names and product names mentioned in this book are subject to trademark, brand or patent protection and are trademarks or registered trademarks of their respective holders. The use of brand names, product names, common names, trade names, product descriptions etc. even without a particular marking in this work is in no way to be construed to mean that such names may be regarded as unrestricted in respect of trademark and brand protection legislation and could thus be used by anyone.

Cover image: www.ingimage.com

This book is a translation from the original published under ISBN 978-613-9-63237-4.

Publisher:
Sciencia Scripts
is a trademark of
Dodo Books Indian Ocean Ltd. and OmniScriptum S.R.L publishing group

120 High Road, East Finchley, London, N2 9ED, United Kingdom
Str. Armeneasca 28/1, office 1, Chisinau MD-2012, Republic of Moldova, Europe
Printed at: see last page
ISBN: 978-620-7-65513-7

I dedicate this work to my parents, who have always encouraged and supported me, for their presence at all times. To Cauã, Giovanna and Carlo, for being part of my life.

ACKNOWLEDGEMENTS

To God, for allowing me to grow personally and professionally during the process of this work, putting wonderful people in my path.

To the coordinator of the Postgraduate Programme in Child and Adolescent Health, Prof. Dr. Mônica Nunes Lima Cat, for her dedication, care and support.

To my supervisor, Dr Adriane Celli, for encouraging me and believing in my work with children with cerebral palsy. For her time, dedication, patience, suggestions and revisions to this study.

To my co-supervisor, speech therapist Dr Edna Marcia Abdulmassih, for her learning, availability, attention, time and dedication.

To Dr Elmar Fugmann and Dr Antonio Ulisses Gavazzoni, for believing in the partnership between speech therapy and otorhinolaryngology, which allowed me to join the Peroral Endoscopy Department at the Hospital de Clínicas of the Federal University of Paraná.

To the Peroral Endoscopy administrative and nursing staff, Renato, Odair, Rosana and Roseli, for their help and patience with our patients.

To the Radiology staff at the Hospital de Clínicas of the Federal University of Paraná, Neno, Lúcia and Eliane, for their care, affection and attention.

To my friends Adriana Betes Heupa, Cristina Muller Sabbag, Gisela Carmona Hirata, Hellen Nathaly Lagos Guimarães and Lilian Messias.

To Professor Rosane Sampaio Santos, for encouraging me to carry out this work.

To all the children with cerebral palsy and their families who took part in this research, who teach me every day the power of love, respect and overcoming.

My great respect and many thanks!

"I don't know if life is short

or too long for us.

But I know that nothing we experience makes sense

if we don't touch people's hearts.

Often it's enough just to be;

A welcoming collar,

Wrapping arm,

A word that comforts;

Silence that respects;

Joy that is contagious;

Tears flowing;

A gaze that caresses;

Desire that satiates;

Love that promotes;

And that's not something out of this world.

It's what gives life meaning.

That's what makes it not even short

Not too long.

But let it be intense, true and pure

While it lasts."

"Happy is he who transfers what he knows

and learns what he teaches."

Cora Coralina

SUMMARY

Dysphagia is a frequent symptom in children with cerebral palsy. Dysphagia associated with the presence of aspiration requires intervention in order to reduce the levels of morbidity and mortality due to recurrent pneumonia and chronic lung diseases. Existing methods for assessing pharyngeal dysphagia are invasive and difficult to access. Non-invasive methods for assessing these patients are needed. The aim of this study was to use Doppler sonography and videofluoroscopy to determine whether there is a significant difference between swallowing sounds in children with and without cerebral palsy. A case-control study was carried out to assess swallowing sounds in 75 children with cerebral palsy and 90 children without neuromotor disorders. The sounds were captured using Doppler sonar simultaneously with videofluoroscopy. Swallowing times were significantly longer in the group of children with cerebral palsy for the two consistencies assessed. There was a significant difference between the two groups for all the variables studied (frequency, intensity and time). Prolonged time in the thick pasty consistency and reduced time in the thin pasty consistency were the acoustic parameters suggestive of risk for aspiration. The data suggests that the swallowing process in patients with cerebral palsy is not only slower than in children without cerebral palsy, but also produces differences in sound patterns that could indicate the presence of oropharyngeal dysphagia, resulting from the abnormalities in muscle tone and movements found in children with this disorder.

Keywords: Swallowing disorders; Doppler sonar: Cerebral Palsy.

SUMMARY

CHAPTER 1

INTRODUCTION

The act of swallowing naturally involves a large number of oral and pharyngeal muscles working together in perfect synchronisation, interrupting breathing and protecting the respiratory tract, a process that normally begins from birth (MARCHESAN, 1999; LOGEMANN, 2007).

When any alteration and/or difficulty in swallowing is observed in the oral cavity, pharynx, oesophagus or oesophagogastric junction, it is called dysphagia and can lead to penetration or aspiration into the respiratory tract, resulting in coughing, suffocation, asphyxia, pulmonary disorders and aspiration pneumonia (SANTINI, 1999; LOGEMANN, 2007).

This difficulty is a frequent symptom in children with cerebral palsy (CP), associated with other complaints such as frequent vomiting, malnutrition, failure to thrive, coughing during and/or after feeding, too long a period of food intake and the presence of pulmonary diseases such as recurrent pneumonia (SANKAR; MUNDKUR, 2005; BAX et al., 2005; AURELIO; GENARO; MACEDO, 2002; FURKIM; BEHLAU; WECKX, 2003).

With regard to dysphagia in children with cerebral palsy, they often have symptoms that include an inability to control food in the mouth, loss of mobility in the upper and lower lips, lack of lip sealing, absence or exacerbation of oral reflexes, early anterior escape, changes in anteroposterior and lateralisation movements of the tongue, changes in the orofacial muscles with loss of intraoral pressure, inadequate propulsion of the food bolus and the presence of intraoral food residue. They may also have pharyngeal alterations, such as a delay in triggering the swallowing reflex, early posterior escape, decreased pharyngeal peristalsis, alterations in laryngeal elevation and contraction, the presence of residue in the epiglottic vallecula and pyriform sinuses and a disturbance in cricopharyngeal muscle motility, with the presence of aspiration before, during or after swallowing (GRIGS; JONES; LEE, 1989; PENNY et al, 1994; WRIGHT; WRIGHT; CARSON,1996; KAHRILA; SHEZLANG; RADEMAKER; LOGEMANN, 1997; GONÇALVES; VIDIGAL, 1999; FURKIM; BEHLAU; WECKX, 2003; MARRARA et al., 2008; KIM; HAN; SONG OH, 2013; ENGEL-HOEK et al., 2014; SU et al., 2016).

The speech therapy clinical assessment combined with the instrumental assessment makes a decisive contribution to defining the necessary clinical, therapeutic or surgical approaches. It consists of an anamnesis carried out with the parents and/or carers with a clinical and neurological history, use of medication, eating routine, complaints and difficulties. It also includes an assessment of the tone, sensitivity and movement of the oral sensorimotor system, a functional assessment of the stomatognathic system, oral reflexes and posture.

The methods currently used to assess, diagnose and monitor dysphagia in children with cerebral palsy include cervical auscultation (EICHER et al., 1995; MCKAIG, 1999; BORR, 2007; FURKIM et al., 2009; LAGARDE; KAMALSKI; ENGEL-HOEK, 2016); nasofibrolaryngoscopy (NFL) (MANRIQUE; MELO; BUHLER, 2002; PAULA et al., 2002) and swallowing studies using videofluoroscopy (VDF) (GRIGS; JONES; LEE, 1989; PENNY et al, 1994; WRIGHT; WRIGHT; CARSON,1996; KAHRILA; SHEZLANG; RADEMAKER; LOGEMANN,1997; GONÇALVES; VIDIGAL, 1999; FURKIM; BEHLAU; WECKX, 2003; MARRARA et al., 2008; KIM; HAN; SONG OH, 2013; ENGEL-HOEK et al., 2014; SU et al., 2016).

The neck region produces a significant amount of acoustic activity and understanding the sounds produced during swallowing is a complex task, which is why cervical auscultation with a stethoscope is a tool for assessing these sounds. Although this technique is non-invasive, its limitations include the lack of standardised measurements and reliance on subjective descriptions of the sounds (FURKIM et al., 2003; CARDOSO; FONTOURA, 2009; BOLZAN et al., 2013; FRAKKING et al., 2013).

Nasofibrolaryngoscopy (NFL) is an invasive test that is not widely accepted in children, as it requires the patient's co-operation and understanding during the test (MANRIQUE; MELO; BUHLER, 2001; MANRIQUE; MELO; BUHLER, 2002; PAULA et al., 2002).

Videofluoroscopy (VDF) is considered the gold standard test for diagnosis, but it has disadvantages such as exposure to radiation, highly trained professionals and rooms with specialised equipment. Furthermore, in Brazil, these studies are generally only carried out in a few tertiary hospitals or specialised clinics, which results in a long waiting list for children who depend on public health services. (ASHA, 2003; FURKIM; BEHLAU; WECKX, 2003; JAFFER et al., 2015).

A non-invasive alternative for assessing swallowing sounds has been used in some studies using Doppler sonar (SANTOS; MACEDO- FILHO, 2006; CAGLIARI; JURKIEWIECZ; SANTOS, 2009; LAGOS, 2013; ABDULMASSIH; TEIVER; SANTOS, 2013; SÓRIA; SILVA; FURKIM, 2016).

The sounds generated as a result of pathological swallowing need to be better identified and the quantification and measurement of these acoustic parameters in a non-invasive way can indicate the presence of pharyngeal dysphagia or aspiration (LAGARDE; KAMALSKI; ENGEL-HOEK, 2015).

1.1. OBJECTIVES

1.1.1   General objective

To evaluate the swallowing sounds of children with and without cerebral palsy, captured by Doppler sonar.

1.1.2   Specific objectives

- Describe the sounds of swallowing in children with and without cerebral palsy;
- To study the role of Doppler sonar in detecting tracheal aspiration.

CHAPTER 2

2.1 DEFINITION OF CEREBRAL PALSY

Cerebral palsy can be defined as:

> A sequela of an encephalic aggression, characterised primarily by a persistent but not invariable disorder of tone, posture and movement, which appears in early childhood and which is not only directly secondary to this non-evolving lesion of the encephalon, but also due to the influence that this lesion exerts on neurological maturation. (KEITH; POLANI,1959, quoted by BAX et al. 2005, p 571).

At the international workshop in Bethesda, Maryland, in 2004, the term cerebral palsy was defined as:

> [...] cerebral palsy (CP) describes a group of disorders of the development of movement and posture, causing activity limitation, that are attributed to non-progressive disturbances that occurred in the developing foetal or infant brain. The motor disorders of cerebral palsy are often accompanied by disturbances of sensation, cognition, communication, perception, behaviour and/or by seizure disorders. (MORRIS, 2007, p. 572).

Cerebral Palsy (CP) is a chronic non-progressive encephalopathy, a neuromotor sequel resulting from complications that occur in the pre-, peri- or post-natal period and can be of congenital, genetic, inflammatory, infectious, anoxic, traumatic or metabolic origin. It occurs very frequently in premature and very low birth weight newborns (NB) due to haemorrhagic lesions in the germinal matrix, which can progress to the ventricular system and/or periventricular white matter (FUNAYAMA; MOURA-RIBEIRO; GONÇALVES, 1997; AURELIO; GENARO; MACEDO-FILHO, 2002; FURKIM; BEHLAU; WECKX, 2003; SANKAR; MUNDKUR, 2005; SILVEIRA; PROCIANOY, 2005).

Extreme premature NBs (under 1500g) often have lung diseases, septicaemia, patent ductus arteriosus and other pathologies that can alter the oxygenation level of the central nervous system. Other pathologies, such as difficult-to-control seizures, hypoglycaemia, hyperbilirubinaemia, meningitis and encephalopathies can also cause cerebral palsy, as can exposure to toxic substances, such as drugs, alcohol, radiation and infectious agents (cytomegalovirus, toxoplasmosis and other).

(AURELIO; GENARO; MACEDO, 2002; FURKIM; BEHLAU; WECKX, 2003; SILVEIRA; PROCIANOY, 2005; KRIGGER, 2006).

2.2 CLASSIFICATION OF CEREBRAL PALSY

Chronic non-progressive encephalopathies of childhood can be classified in various ways. It can take into account the time and place of the lesion, the aetiology, the symptomatology or the topographical distribution. As for classification, it can traditionally be based on the anatomical and clinical aspects of cerebral palsy, being divided into quadriplegia, hemiplegia and diplegia (MINEAR, 1956; ROTTA, 2002; BOBATH, 2000; PAULSON; VARGUS-ADAMS, 2017).

When classified according to motor system: as spastic, hypotonic, ataxic, dyskinetic (athetoid and dystonic) and mixed; in topographical distribution: as quadriplegic, hemiplegic and diplegic (ROTTA, 2002; BOBATH, 2000; PAULSON; VARGUS-ADAMS, 2017).

The Gross Motor Function Classification *System* (GMFCS), proposed by Palisano et al. (1997), assesses the severity of the child's neuromotor sequelae in five levels, graded from I to V, with I being total independence of mobility and locomotion up to level V being total dependence on the carer (PAULSON; VARGUS-ADAMS, 2017).

The *Manual Ability Classification System* (MACS) developed by Eliasson *et al.* (2006), complements the GMFCS, aimed at children aged 4 to 18 with cerebral palsy to assess manual function and fine motor control, with a classification scale, also in 5 levels, graduated from I to V, with level I as manual skills without limitations and/or difficulties up to V with total manual inability, need for support, assistance and adapted equipment. (PAULSON; VARGUS-ADAMS, 2017).

The *Communication Function Classification System* (CFCS) was developed by Hidecker *et al.* (2011), as a complement to the GMFCS and MACS, to assess the communication of children with cerebral palsy in terms of comprehension and expression, also classified into 5 levels, graded from I to V, level I being related to effective communication, without the need for assistance, up to V ineffective communication. (HIDECKER et al., 2011; PAULSON; VARGUS-ADAMS, 2017).

The Eating and Drinking Ability Classification System (EDACS) developed by Sellers et al. (2014), also complements the GMFCS, MACS and CFCS for the feeding capacity of children with cerebral palsy over 3 years of age, assessing food safety to avoid aspiration and asphyxia, with indications of the amount of food ingested, time used during feeding, verifying the need for assistance from the responsible person or carer, level I is related to independence during feeding, with food safety and efficiency for different consistencies and textures, up to level V, which indicates a risk of aspiration, with a ban on oral ingestion, suggesting feeding via gastrostomy. (PAULSON; VARGUS-ADAMS, 2017; BENFER et al, 2017).

When considering functionality, the Paediatric Evaluation of Disability Inventory (PEDI) classifies motor impairment into levels of severity according to limitations and the need to use assistive technology, assessing children's capacity, ability and functional performance through an interview with the carer, which involves 197 items, subdivided into: mobility (59 items, involving use of the bathroom, bathing and the possibility of using stairs), self-care (73 items) and social function (65 items). Each item is scored on its ability or inability to perform and there is also an assessment of the carer's assistance on a scale of 1 to 5 (MANRIQUE; MELO; BUHLER, 2002; CHAGAS et al., 2007; VIVONE et al., 2007; VASCONCELOS et al., 2009).

Currently, the International Classification of Functioning, Disability and Health (ICF), approved by the World Health Organisation, has been more widely used to assess the functional performance of children with cerebral palsy, focusing on health limitations and impairment in carrying out daily activities. It is subdivided into two components: the area of functionality and disability (body functions and structure, activities and participation) and environmental and personal factors, with each component containing several domains and each domain several categories (BRASILEIRO et al., 2009).

2.3 THE CHILD WITH CEREBRAL PALSY

Children with cerebral palsy may have changes in neuromotor function, anatomically classified as quadriplegia, diplegia and various paresis and/or changes in oral motor function, which are also common (AURELIO; GENARO; MACEDO, 2002; FURKIM; BEHLAU; WECKX, 2003; SILVEIRA; PROCIANOY, 2005; KRIGGER, 2006). There may also be other associated alterations, such as cognitive impairment, sensory deficits (visual or auditory) and seizures. Children with quadriplegia have major oral motor and sensory difficulties, with altered cervical control, exacerbated reflexes and/or reduced sensitivity, which affects the entire swallowing process (AURELIO; GENARO; MACEDO-FILHO, 2002; MANRIQUE; MELO; BUHLER, 2002; FURKIM; BEHLAU; WECKX, 2003; KRIGGER, 2006; CHAGAS et al., 2007; VIVONE et al., 2007).

Altered oral motor function, with the presence of dysphagia, has been reported on a daily basis by parents and/or carers as one of the major problems faced by children with cerebral palsy, as well as other complaints such as frequent vomiting, malnutrition, altered weight and height growth, coughing and choking during or after feeding, very long food intake times, refusal to eat, eating a small amount of food and the presence of lung problems with recurrent pneumonia. (ROTTA, 2002; AURELIO; GENARO; MACEDO-FILHO, 2002; FURKIM et al, 2003; CHAGAS et al., 2008; VIANA; SUZUKI, 2011; KIM et al., 2013).

2.4 NORMAL SWALLOWING

Swallowing can be divided into two voluntary phases (preparatory and oral) and two involuntary phases (pharyngeal and oesophageal). The oral preparatory phase begins with the capture of the food bolus, lip sealing, lateralisation of the tongue to move the food bolus between the teeth to grind and chew the food, preparing it for swallowing, with rotatory movements of the mandible and sensory perception of the tongue, in order to initiate anteroposterior movements that propel the food bolus into the oropharynx. The oropharyngeal phase then begins, with closure of the velopharynx in order to prevent food from escaping into the nasal cavity, triggering the swallowing reflex, the sequence of laryngeal elevation and contraction, closure of the epiglottis and the true and false vocal folds, movement of the tongue base and opening of the cricopharynx, thus directing the food bolus into the oesophagus. This allows the oesophageal phase of swallowing to continue. This whole process takes place quickly, in around two to three seconds (LOGEMANN, 2007).

2.5 SWALLOWING IN CHILDREN WITH CEREBRAL PALSY

Altered oral motor function, with the presence of dysphagia, has been reported by parents and carers as one of the biggest problems for children with cerebral palsy, accompanied by complaints such as frequent vomiting, malnutrition, growth deficit, coughing during and/or after feeding and the presence of pulmonary disorders with recurrent pneumonia.

According to Padovani (2007) dysphagia is a swallowing disorder resulting from neurological and/or structural causes. Dysphagia often reflects problems involving the oral cavity, pharynx, oesophagus or oesophagogastric transition, which can lead to food entering the airways, resulting in coughing, choking, asphyxia, lung problems and aspiration. It can also lead to nutritional deficits and dehydration with consequent weight loss.

A large percentage of children with cerebral palsy have oropharyngeal dysphagia with an inability to control food in the mouth, difficulty sealing the lips, early loss of food, loss and/or presence of exacerbated oral reflexes, lack of control over tongue movement, altered orofacial muscles with decreased intraoral pressure, delayed triggering of the swallowing reflex, pharyngeal leak, decreased pharyngeal peristalsis and aspiration before, during or after swallowing, as well as altered laryngeal elevation. (ROGERS et al., 1994; ARVEDSON et al., 1994; SANTINI,1999; PENNY et al., 1994; AURELIO; GENARO; MACEDO, 2002; MANRIQUE. MELO. BUHLER, 2002; MANRIQUE, 2003; FURKIM. BEHLAU.

WECKX, 2003; LOGEMAN, 2007; VIVONE et al., 2007; CHAGAS et al., 2008; VIANA; SUZUKI, 2011; ARAUJO; SILVA; MENDES, 2012; ARVEDSON, 2013).

2.6 CLASSIFICATION OF DYSPHAGIA

According to Ott et al. (1996) dysphagia can be classified as: a) Normal swallowing; b) Mild dysphagia: when there is altered oral control, with delayed pharyngeal response, presence of little residue, no penetration or laryngotracheal aspiration; c) Moderate dysphagia: with poor oral control, presence of pharyngeal residue in all consistencies, little penetration or laryngotracheal aspiration of one consistency; d) Severe dysphagia: with substantial laryngotracheal aspiration. (OTT et al, 1996).

According to the Severity Rating Scale, swallowing can be categorised as:

> a) Normal swallowing: the presence of movements and coordination are appropriate for the age group and according to the type of food offered. b) Swallowing with mild impairment: when it is identified, but functional, with anteroposterior movements, with a possible delay in the swallowing reflex; with slow transit of the food through the pharynx, with a possible presence of some residues, but with a protective cough in the event of a small penetration of the food into the respiratory cavity. c) Swallowing with moderate impairment: the preparation of the food bolus is slow, with inadequate movement of the bolus in the oral cavity, with little efficiency and a delay in the swallowing reflex, with residues remaining in the oral cavity and throughout swallowing and requiring multiple swallows, with the presence of aspiration and/or silent aspiration. d) Severely impaired swallowing: little or no oral movement, presence of sialorrhoea, anterior loss of most of the food bolus, delayed triggering of the swallowing reflex, residues in the pyriform sinuses, reduced pharyngeal peristalsis and aspiration in all textures and consistencies, in which case oral feeding is contraindicated (PENNY et al., 1994), 1994).

2.7 CLINICAL ASSESSMENT OF SWALLOWING IN CHILDREN WITH CEREBRAL PALSY

The swallowing assessment should include an anamnesis, which should be carried out with parents and/or carers, and include an investigation of personal history, to identify the etiology of the neurological alteration, the use of medication, the child's daily and eating routine, and the main complaints and difficulties. Clinical assessment of the structures of the stomatognathic system involved in the feeding process should include analysing tone, mobility and the presence or absence of oral and global reflexes, as well as clinical assessment of the teeth, mandible, hard palate, soft palate, tongue, pharynx, voice, level of attention and the use or need for adaptations. (QUINTELLA; SILVA, 1999; GROHER, 1999; GONÇALVES; VIDIGAL, 1999; FURKIM; BEHLAU; WECKX; 2003; LOGEMAN, 2007; FURKIM et al, 2009, VIANA; SUZUKI, 2011).

2.8 INSTRUMENTAL ASSESSMENT OF SWALLOWING

To assess, diagnose and monitor dysphagia in children with cerebral palsy, the NFL (MANRIQUE; MELO; BUHLER; 2002), VDF of swallowing (GRIGS; JONES; LEE, 1989; PENNY et al., 1994; ARVEDSON et al., 1994; WRIGHT; WRIGHT; CARSON, 1996; KAHRILA et al, 1997; GONÇALVES; VIDIGAL, 1999; FURKIM; BEHLAU; WECKX, 2003; MARRARA et al., 2008;

KIM; HAN; SONG OH; 2013; ENGEL-HOEK et al., 2014; SU et al., 2016) and cervical auscultation (MCKAIG, 1999; FURKIM; DUARTE; SACCA; SÓRIA, 2009). More recently, Doppler sonar has been used in various studies to analyse the acoustic sounds of swallowing and dysphagia in different pathologies (SANTOS; MACEDO-FILHO, 2006; CAGLIARI; JURKIEWICZ; SANTOS; MARQUES, 2009; LAGOS et al., 2013; ABDULMASSIH, 2013; SÓRIA; SILVA; FURKIM, 2016).

Logeman (2007) emphasised the importance of knowing the underlying disease that causes dysphagia, as well as its pathophysiology. The swallowing alterations that each patient presents must be properly analysed for individualised therapeutic planning, with more efficient and safer results.

2.8.1 Nasofibrolaryngoscopy

In this instrumental assessment of swallowing, a fiberscope is introduced into one of the nostrils, using food with blue aniline for structural and functional assessment of the nasal fossae, rhinopharynx, velopharyngeal sphincter, tongue base, vallecula, lateral and posterior pharyngeal walls, piriform recesses and larynx. It also assesses the presence or absence of stasis and aspiration during the swallowing process (MANRIQUE; MELO; BUHLER, 2001; MANRIQUE; MELO; BUHLER, 2002; PAULA et al., 2002).

2.8.2 Videofluoroscopy

The dynamic study of swallowing by VDF is considered the gold standard test for assessing dysphagia. Through VDF, the speech therapist assesses the anatomical structures of the mouth, pharynx, oesophagus and cervical region and checks for possible abnormalities in the lips, tongue, palate, teeth, mandible, soft palate, epiglottis, vallecula, pyriform sinuses, hyoid, larynx, trachea, upper oesophageal sphincter (cricopharyngeal) and cervical spine. The VDF makes it possible to assess the physiology of swallowing and observe the ability to control and move food in the mouth, lip closure ability and its efficiency, the presence of extraoral escape, oral reflexes, movement of the anterior part and dorsum of the tongue, tongue control, escape into the rhinopharynx, early posterior escape, swallowing reflex, laryngeal elevation and contraction. It also makes it possible to assess content clearance, the presence of stasis in the vallecula and pyriform sinuses, oesophageal emptying, the presence of airway penetration and aspiration before, during or after swallowing, airway protection, the presence or absence of efficient coughing, the need for multiple swallows, the functioning of the upper oesophageal sphincter and the presence of gastro-oesophageal reflux. (ASHA, 2003; FURKIM; BEHLAU; WECKX, 2003; JAFFER et al, 2015).

The VDF also allows changes in posture, movements or compensatory manoeuvres that facilitate swallowing to be visualised in real time and can provide patients and family members with individualised guidance and care during feeding, preventing aspiration (ASHA, 2003; FURKIM; BEHLAU; WECKX, 2003; LOGEMAN, 2007; JAFFER et al., 2015).

Several authors have carried out research and studies on swallowing in children and adolescents with cerebral palsy using the VDF of swallowing (GRIGS; JONES; LEE, 1989; PENNY et al., 1994; WRIGHT; WRIGHT; CARSON, 1996; FURKIM, BEHLAU; WECKX, 2003; DE MATTEO; MATOVICH; HJARTASON, 2005;

MARRARA et al., 2008; KIM; HAN; SONG OH, 2013; ENGEL-HOEK et al., 2014; SU et al., 2016; LAGOS-GUIMARÃES et al., 2016).

Compared to clinical speech assessment, instrumental assessment of swallowing by VDF in children with spastic tetraparetic cerebral palsy makes it possible to identify silent aspiration, which is quite common in this situation. Chronic aspirators can desensitise the larynx and stop coughing after a long period of aspiration. Therefore, after clinical assessment, when there is a possibility of silent aspiration or a risk of aspiration, CDV is used as a complementary assessment to investigate dysphagia in children and adolescents with cerebral palsy (GRIGS; JONES; LEE, 1989; PENNY et al, 1994; WRIGHT; WRIGHT; CARSON, 1996; NEWMANN et al., 2001; FURKIM; BEHLAU; WECKX, 2003; MARRARA et al., 2008; WEIR et al., 2011; KIM; HAN; SONG OH, 2013; ENGEL-HOEK et al., 2014; BAE et al., 2014; SU et al., 2016).

2.8.3 Cervical auscultation

The neck region produces a significant amount of acoustic activity and understanding sound production during swallowing has been a complex task for several authors who have dedicated themselves to the subject in recent decades. Although cervical auscultation is non-invasive, its limitations include the lack of standardised measurements and reliance on subjective descriptions of sounds (CARDOSO; FONTOURA, 2009; BOLZAN et al., 2013; LAGARDE; KAMALSKI; ENGEL-HOEK, 2015).

Cervical auscultation is a non-invasive procedure that is useful for assessing and analysing oropharyngeal coordination and the respiratory pause required during food intake. It analyses the synchrony between sucking/mastication, respiratory pause and swallowing, and whether or not laryngotracheal aspiration occurs during this event, using a stethoscope as a sound amplification instrument. Some studies have also used a microphone and accelerometer (FRAKKING et al., 2013; LAGARDE; KAMALSKI; ENGEL-HOEK, 2015).

The authors Hamlet, Nelson and Patterson (1990) described a theory on the physiological cause of the origin of swallowing sounds and emphasised that the most prominent acoustic characteristic of the swallowing sound corresponds to the movement of the bolus in the pharynx and upper oesophageal sphincter. They stated that a periodic noise, perhaps of laryngeal origin, "explodes" as the cricopharyngeus muscle closes. Hyoid, laryngeal and epiglottic movement also contribute to the acoustic signal of swallowing.

Takahashi, Groher and Michi (1994) studied the best location for analysing and acoustically perceiving swallowing. They also analysed the best adhesive for fixation and the best acoustic detector for capturing swallowing sounds. The accelerometer with a double strip showed the best results for capturing the sound signal of swallowing and the lateral edge of the trachea, immediately below the cricoid cartilage, was the best location for capturing the sounds of swallowing, with the best signal-to-noise ratio and the lowest variance, avoiding the joint capture of blood circulation in the carotid artery.

Thus, based on this theory, normal swallowing consists of an audible double click and three additional components are responsible for the sound produced during swallowing. The first corresponds to a weak signal associated with the elevation and forward excursion of the larynx, as well as the passage of the bolus through the pharynx; the second is a strong sound associated with the opening of the upper cricopharyngeal sphincter and the third a weak signal associated with the descent of the larynx after swallowing. (LAGARDE; KAMALSKI; ENGEL-HOEK, 2016; HAMLET; NELSON; PATTERSON, 1990; HAMLET; PATTERSON; FLEMING; JONES, 1992; CICHERO; MURDOCH, 1998).

Several researchers have studied the acoustic characteristics of swallowing using cervical auscultation in babies, children and adults with and without dysphagia (BORR et al., 2007; CARDOSO; FONTOURA, 2009; FURKIM et al., 2009; FRAKKING et al., 2013; BOLZAN et al., 2013; SILVA, 2013; TAMANINI, 2013). Other non-invasive procedures used to assess normal and pathological swallowing, based on swallowing sounds, have already been described and included the use of an accelerometer and microphone (EICHER et al., 1995; MCKAIG, 1999; LESLIE et al., 2007; FURKIM et al., 2009; PATATAS et al., 2011). Jestrovi et al. (2013) and Hammoudi et al. (2014) carried out studies of swallowing sounds in normal individuals to observe differences in the bolus and viscosity of the food.

2.8.   4Cervical auscultation   with Doppler sonar

Taylor (1988) initially reported the use of Doppler sonar to capture foetal sounds, in which ultrasound pulses are transmitted to the patient's body. The sound wave can be captured through the vibration that occurs in material media, with moments of compression and rarefaction of the medium, with the structures returning to their resting position (MCKAIG; STROUD, 1996).

Doppler sonar equipment used in healthcare has ultrasound transducers with piezoelectric ceramic materials to generate and detect sound waves. The transducer transforms electrical energy into ultrasonic energy, emitting and capturing the echo signals that have been sent out by the moments of compression and rarefaction of the medium (ZAGZEBSKI, 1996).

A computer with appropriate software for acoustic analysis digitises the swallowing sounds captured and transforms them into sound waves, enabling a more precise analysis (SPADOTTO et al., 2008; SPADOTTO et al., 2012).

Based on the theories of cervical auscultation to assess swallowing sounds, Santos and Macedo-Filho (2006) proposed analysing swallowing sounds with the Doppler sonar instrument and suggested, in a study of 50 normal individuals, the feasibility of its use for diagnosis and therapeutic monitoring of dysphagia. The study method made it possible to trace the normality pattern of the sound of swallowing using Doppler sonar, analysing time and acoustic frequency. The same parameters were also studied in 90 healthy children by Cagliari et al. (2009):

> The Doppler effect is defined as the change in frequency sensation resulting from a situation in which the sound source is mobile, travelling at a constant speed, and the receiver is stationary at some point along its path. As the sound source approaches the receiver, it receives a greater number of waves per unit time (higher frequency) and as it moves away it receives a smaller number of waves (lower frequency). In continuous Doppler, the emitted signal can be represented by a continuous sinusoid, whose amplitude is associated with the pressure variation in the propagation medium or the displacement of the particles. The computer is able to digitise the sounds and process the noises produced by swallowing into waveform visual representations (CAGLIARI et al., 2009, p. 707).

In 2016, Sória, Silva and Furkim studied swallowing sounds in healthy young and elderly adults to analyse sound patterns and their relationship with ageing. Abdulmassih, Teive and Santos, in 2013, compared the signals

analysed the acoustic parameters of swallowing in adults with and without spinocerebellar ataxia. Lagos et al., 2013, analysed the acoustic parameters of swallowing in newborn babies. There are no other studies evaluating swallowing sounds with Doppler sonar in children with dysphagia.

The instrumental assessment that complements the clinical examination makes a decisive contribution to defining the clinical, therapeutic and, when necessary, surgical approaches to be taken. According to Furkim, Behlau and Weckx (2003) and Logeman (2007), speech therapists are concerned with drawing up an appropriate and individualised therapeutic plan for treating patients with dysphagia and detecting bronchoaspiration during the feeding process.

The dynamic study of swallowing using FDV may be the most detailed, but it exposes the patient to radiation and so cannot be prolonged, and there are still few specialised venues that carry out this examination (BOLZAN et al., 2013).

The sounds generated during swallowing can be used as an aid in the clinical diagnosis of swallowing, but more studies of non-invasive methods are needed in order to correctly standardise, assess and analyse the sounds considered to be adequate or pathological (indicators of dysphagia).

CHAPTER 3

MATERIAL AND METHODS

3.1 TYPE OF STUDY

This is an observational, analytical, case-control, ambispective study, retrospective for the control group and prospective for the study group.

3.2 STUDY HYPOTHESIS

Acoustic parameters make it possible to identify children with oropharyngeal dysphagia.

3.3 PLACE AND PERIOD OF STUDY

The clinical assessment was carried out in the Per-Oral Endoscopy department and in the Neuropediatrics outpatient clinic at the Hospital de Clínicas de Curitiba, using the swallowing clinical assessment protocol already used by this department (Appendix 1). Children were referred for assessment according to demand from the Regional Centre for the Care of the Disabled (CRAID), special schools and the gastro-pediatrics, child neurology (CENEP), neonatal and paediatric ICU sectors.

The VDF was carried out in the Peri-oral Radiology and Endoscopy department of the Hospital de Clínicas de Curitiba of the Federal University of Paraná, based on the swallowing assessment protocol already used by this department (Appendix 2).

Data collection began in May 2010 and was finalised in May 2015, with some periods of interruption due to the unavailability of the videofluoroscope.

3. 4SOURCE POPULATION

The source population was made up of children diagnosed with cerebral palsy who complained of dysphagia and were referred to the per-oral endoscopy department for a dynamic swallowing study by VDF, with an average of 72 children per year.

3.5   INCLUSION CRITERIA

  a)   Study group
-   Children whose parents or guardians have signed the Free and Informed Consent Form (FICF) (Appendix 1);
-          Both sexes from 0 to 15 years old;
-          Diagnosed with cerebral palsy;
-          Complains of difficulty eating;
-          Alert and responsive when offered food;
-          With oropharyngeal dysphagia.

  b)   Control Group
-   Children whose parents or guardians have signed the Informed Consent Form (ICF, Appendix 1);
-   Both sexes from 2 to 15 years old;
-   Alert and responsive when offered food;
-   With normal swallowing.

3.6   EXCLUSION CRITERIA

  a)   Study Group
-   Child forbidden to eat orally.
-   With structural changes in the head and neck.
-   Refusal or inability to swallow at least 1 consistency (liquid, thin pasty and thick pasty).

-With constant crying during the Doppler sonar evaluation; this data was excluded after acoustic analysis.

  b)   Control group
-   Refusal or inability to swallow at least 1 consistency (saliva, liquid and thin pasty);
-Constant crying during the Doppler sonar evaluation; this data was excluded after acoustic analysis.

3.   7STUDY POPULATION

Given the inclusion and exclusion criteria, 165 children made up the study population, 75 from the study group and 90 from the control group. The data on the acoustic parameters of the swallowing of the 90 children in the control group is part of a study carried out previously by researcher Cibele Fontoura Cagliari, who provided this data for a comparative study.

3. 8STUDY VARIABLES

The variables studied were the acoustic parameters of swallowing (initial frequency, peak frequency, final frequency, initial intensity, peak intensity, final intensity and time) with the food consistencies liquid, thin pasty (nectar) and thick pasty (pudding).

3. 9STUDY PROCEDURES

3.9. 1Clinical assessment

The clinical assessment consisted of an anamnesis with parents and/or carers, followed by an assessment of the oral sensory-motor system, checking mobility and tone,

sensitivity and oral reflexes. Subsequently, an instrumental assessment of swallowing was carried out using VDF and Doppler sonar (Appendices 1, 2 and 3).

Swallowing sounds were recorded simultaneously with the VDF in order to analyse swallowing and breathing coordination. We also checked for possible noises or sound signals that might indicate laryngeal penetration or aspiration.

3.3.1 Videofluoroscopy

Siemens Axiom model R100® and Siemens monitor M44-2® X-ray machines were used to carry out the videofluoroscopic swallowing study. The images were digitised on the HP Pavilion TX 2075BR® notebook, using the Sapphire Wonder TV® USB TV capture card.

During the assessment, the children remained seated with the support of a car seat, comfort baby or adapted chair, adjusted to 90 degrees, with a lateral radiographic view, keeping the neck region free (PENNY et al., 1994; ASHA, 2003; FURKIM; BEHLAU; WECKX, 2003; MARRARA et al., 2008; ARVEDSON, 2013; JAFFER et al., 2015). We chose the lateral region of the trachea, immediately below the cricoid cartilage, on the right side, as the best adaptation of the transducer and the best sound signal collection (TAKAHASHI; GROHER; MICHI; 1994).

Contact gel was used to facilitate adherence of the transducer to the skin, to favour acoustic signal capture and avoid interference.

The food consistencies offered during the VDF and capture of swallowing sounds with the Doppler sonar were nectar (thin puree), pudding (thickened puree) and liquid, according to the nomenclature of the American Dietetic Association, as well as according to the Guidelines of Speech-Language Pathologists Performing Videofluoroscopic Swallowing Studies (ASHA, 2003) and Swallowing and Swallowing Disorders (Dysphagia). To obtain these consistencies, 70% water was used mixed with 100% barium sulphate (Bariogel® - radiological contrast containing 1g of barium sulphate and 1ml of gsp vehicle for paediatric and adult use) and an instant food thickener (Thick&Easy® - composed of modified corn starch - E1442, maltodextrin, tara gum, xanthan gum and guar gum, with a nutritional composition of 100g, 375kcal, 100g of carbohydrates and 125mg of sodium. The recipe and consistency indications were used according to the manufacturer's instructions.

The child was offered 5ml of each consistency (a dessert spoon), with at least three swallows of each consistency offered, which were observed and recorded during a 2-minute interval (ASHA, 2003). Disposable cups, spoons, plastic syringes and, when necessary, the child's own bottle were used as utensils to offer the food. A quantity of 5ml was stipulated to ensure the quantity was appropriate for young children, as well as older children, since the age difference varied greatly.

No solid food was offered during VDF and Doppler sonar testing due to the great difficulty in feeding the children in the study group (children with quadriplegia and oropharyngeal dysphagia, with no functional chewing pattern, whose parents and/or carers reported that the children were not used to and/or did not accept eating solid food).

In addition to the researcher/speech therapist and the teacher/volunteer experienced in carrying out the VDF exam, a radiologist was present to check the equipment, adjusting the dosage and time of exposure to radiation. The mother, father or guardian who accompanied the child during the examination usually helped with the contrasted food, mentioning food preferences, consistencies offered daily and care used during feeding.

Appropriate safety equipment was used during the VDF examinations, such as a lead apron and thyroid protector, goggles and disposable gloves for offering the barium contrasted food, by the professionals and parents accompanying the examination.

DFV was carried out in a hospital environment and no cases with complications or requiring emergency procedures were recorded.

The examination includes a structural and anatomical assessment of the lips, teeth, jaw, hard palate, soft palate, tongue, pharynx, larynx, epiglottis, upper oesophageal sphincter and oesophagus.

During the swallowing assessment, lip closure, anterior escape or extraoral escape, the presence of multiple swallows, sufficient or insufficient bolus formation, prolonged oral time, decreased tongue movement and the presence of residue in the oral cavity were observed in the oral phase. During the pharyngeal phase, we considered the delayed onset of pharyngeal swallowing, early posterior escape, oral ejection into the pharynx, contrast passing through the pharynx, pharyngeal residue (vallecula and pyriform sinuses), hyoid movement, laryngeal penetration and tracheal aspiration. The disorders that were analysed and observed involving the pharyngeal phase included a delayed or absent swallowing reflex, inadequate laryngeal contraction and/or elevation, penetration or aspiration before, during or after swallowing. Protection of the upper airways was also assessed, with elevation and anteriorisation of the larynx and closure of the epiglottis. Laryngeal penetration and tracheal aspiration were carefully assessed before, during and after swallowing.

The assessment of the oesophageal phase considered oesophageal peristalsis, the opening of the lower oesophageal sphincter (cricopharyngeal) and the presence of gastro-oesophageal reflux.

The characteristics of VDF were classified according to the severity of dysphagia, as described by Ott et al. (1996), into mild, moderate or severe dysphagia. When there is difficulty in oral control, delayed pharyngeal response, presence of little residue and no penetration or tracheal aspiration, dysphagia can be classified as mild. Poor oral control, presence of pharyngeal residues in all consistencies and little tracheal penetration or aspiration of one consistency correspond to moderate dysphagia, while severe dysphagia is associated with substantial tracheal aspiration. The VDF images were recorded simultaneously with the swallowing sounds captured by the Doppler sonar.

The parents and/or guardians of the children who took part in the VDF and Doppler sonar assessment received the report with the opinion of the instrumental assessment of swallowing using VDF.

3.9.3 Sonar   Doppler

The equipment used to carry out the Doppler sonar swallowing study was a Martec® DF-4001 Ultrasonic Detector (portable), with a single crystal flat disc transducer as the Doppler interface. The Doppler ultrasound frequency is 2.5 MHz, with an output of 10 mW/cm^2 . The sound output power is 1W.

The Doppler sonar equipment was attached to a notebook and the acoustic signals of the swallowing sounds were recorded and then analysed using version 2.8 of the VoxMetria software (developed by CTS Computers®) by Behlau and Michaelis (2003), enabling precise measurement.

This software is capable of processing the noise produced by swallowing and representing it visually in wave format, in order to analyse intensity, frequency and time (Figure 1).

The Doppler sonar transducer was placed on the right side of the neck, in the lateral portion of the trachea, just below the cricoid cartilage, as described by Takahashi, Groher and Michi (1994) as the best place for cervical auscultation, as illustrated in Figure 2. The ultrasonic energy beam emitted by the transducer was positioned to form an angle of 30°-60°. In order to reduce the dispersion of the ultrasound into the air and increase its transmission through the body and echo, Contact® gel was used, favouring the recording of the acoustic signal for later analysis (TAKAHASHI; GROHER; MICHI; 1994; YOUMANSS; STIERWALT, 2005).

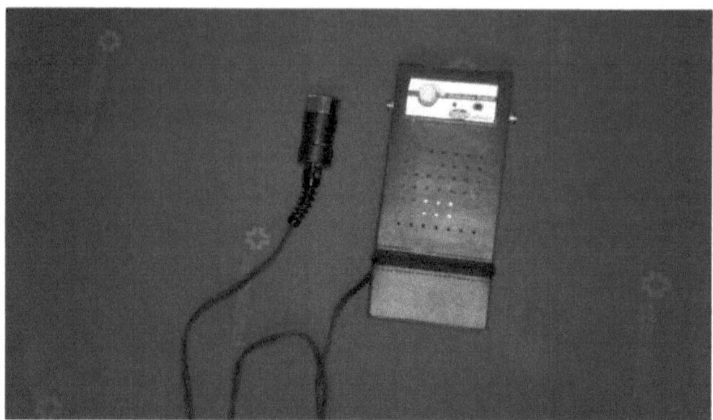

FIGURA 1- DOPPLER SONAR EQUIPMENT USED DURING THE RESEARCH TO CAPTURE SWALLOWING SOUNDS

SOURCE: The author (2017)

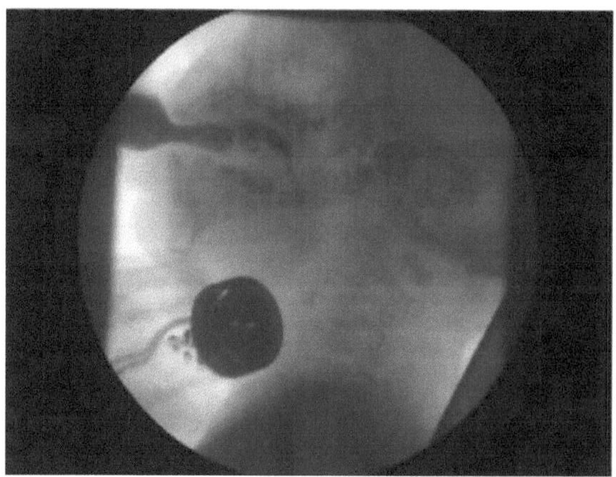

FIGURA 2- POSITIONING THE DOPPLER SONAR TO CAPTURE SWALLOWING SOUNDS **CONCOMITANTLY WITH THE VDF** - DEMONSTRATION OF THE ORAL PHASE, WITH LIQUID SUCTION FROM A BOTTLE, A CHILD WITH CEREBRAL PALSY AND OROPHARYNGEAL DYSPHAGIA

SOURCE: The author (2017).

24

After recording each child's name, date of birth, age and date of assessment, the researcher created a sound file for later analysis, for each consistency. The software's voice analysis function was chosen to record the swallowing sound using the following parameters: audio signal, intensity and

fundamental frequency. The volume of the Doppler sonar device was set to number 1 for a better audio signal, allowing for a "cleaner" signal and avoiding interference from external noise, for later analysis using VoxMetria (Figure 3).

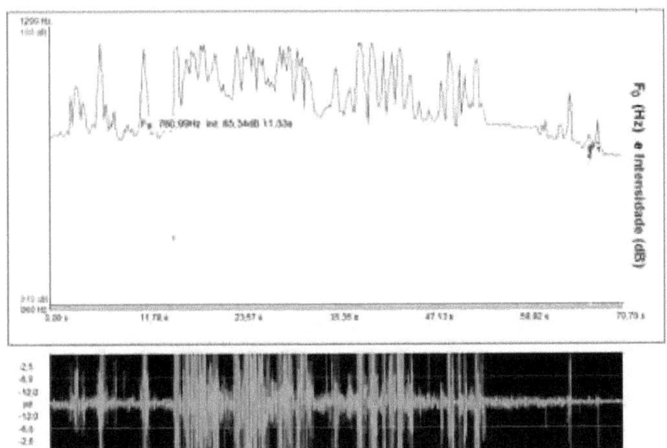

FIGURE 3- SOUND CURVE AND SPECTROGRAM FROM VOXMETRIA *SOFTWARE* CAPTURED DURING VDF AND DOPPLER SONAR - A FILE WAS CREATED FOR EACH CONSISTENCY
SOURCE: Voxmetria

The data from the acoustic signals of swallowing in this study were analysed and classified as previously described by Santos and Macedo (2006) and Abdulmassih et al. (2013):

a) Initial Frequency (IF) of the sound wave - frequency at the start of the acoustic process signal, measured in Hz.

b) Peak Frequency (PF) of the sound wave - frequency of the highest point of displacement of the acoustic signal, measured in Hz.

c) Final Frequency (FF) - frequency at the end of the sound curve, measured in Hz.

d) Initial Intensity (II) - initial intensity of the acoustic signal recorded by the Doppler sonar during the swallowing event, ranging from 10dB to 140dB.

e) Peak Intensity (PI) - peak of the wave recorded by the Doppler sonar during the swallowing event, amplitude of the sound signal ranging from 10dB to 140dB.

f)   Final Intensity (IF) - final intensity of the acoustic signal of the sound wave.

25

g) Swallowing time (T) - time elapsed from swallowing apnoea to laryngeal descent after post-swallowing expiration, completing the full swallowing cycle, from the beginning to the end of the acoustic signal, measured in seconds (Figure 4).

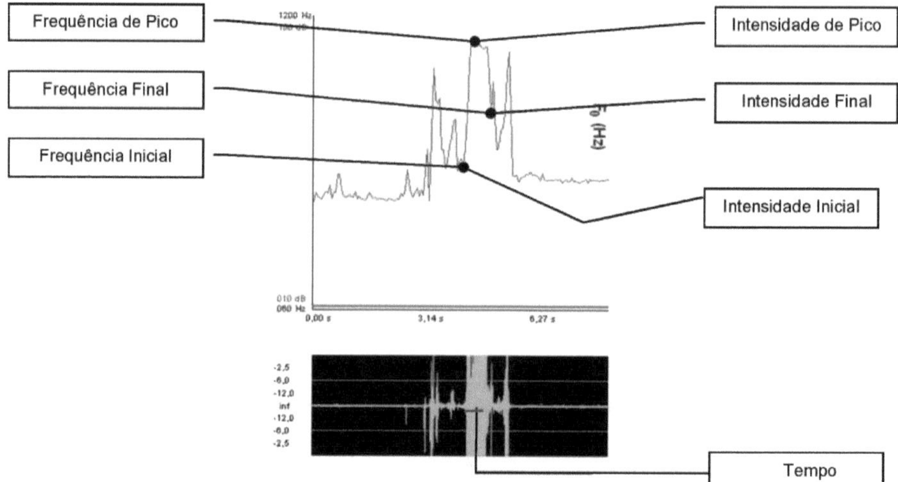

FIGURE 4- GRAPHIC REPRESENTATION OF SWALLOWING SOUND VARIABLES CAPTURED BY DOPPLER SONAR
SOURCE: Adapted from Abdulmassih (2013).

The numbers 1, 2 and 3 have been added to the abbreviations of the above variables to represent the consistencies, respectively, as follows: FI1, FP1, FF1, II1, IP1, IF1, T1 for these variables during swallowing of the liquid consistency; FI2, FP2, FF2, II2, IP2, IF2, T2 for these variables during swallowing of the nectar consistency; FI3, FP3, FF3, II3, IP3, IF3, T3 for these variables during swallowing of the pudding consistency. Figure 4 shows the graphical representation of the variables (initial, peak and final frequency, initial, peak and final intensity, swallowing time) for the two groups studied using Doppler sonar. The best audio and video sample from each child was selected to analyse the frequency, intensity and duration of swallowing. The association between swallowing sound signals and anatomical structural movements observed in the VDF, according to studies already described by Morinière (2008), are shown in Table 1.

CHART 1 - CORRELATION BETWEEN ACOUSTIC SWALLOWING SIGNALS AND THE MOVEMENT OF ANATOMICAL STRUCTURES OBSERVED DURING VIDEOFLUOROSCOPY

ACOUSTIC SIGNS OF SWALLOWING (DOPPLER)	ANATOMICAL STRUCTURES (VFSS)
Initial Frequency (IF) and Initial Intensity (II)	Elevation of the larynx (beginning of the pharyngeal phase of swallowing)
Peak Frequency (PF) and Peak Intensity (PI)	Opening of the cricopharyngeus muscle (upper oesophageal sphincter)
Final Frequency (FF) and Final Intensity	Return of structures (descent of the larynx)

(IF)	
Time (T)	Elapsed time from start to end of acoustic signal

SOURCE: Adapted from Morinière (2008)

3.10 TABULATION AND DATA MANAGEMENT

The data collected during the clinical assessment was recorded on a data collection form drawn up by the author (Appendix 1) and then entered into an Excel spreadsheet (Microsoft®).

The VDF images were recorded on the computer and analysed at least 3 times for each child assessed.

Acoustic swallowing data was recorded and then analysed for each consistency swallowed by the child.

All the data was collected and analysed by the researcher under the supervision of her co-supervisor, Professor Edna M. da Silva Abdulmassih, a specialist in VDF.

3.11 STATISTICAL ANALYSIS

Statistica 10.0 software (Statsoft®) was used to analyse the data. Continuous variables are expressed as mean and standard deviation and median, minimum and maximum values. Categorical variables are expressed as absolute and relative frequencies. Student's t-test and ANOVA with Duncan's post-hoc test were used to estimate the difference between continuous variables with a symmetrical distribution. For asymmetrically distributed variables, the Mann-Whitney and Kruskal-Wallis ANOVA tests were used. Estimates of differences between categorical variables were analysed using Fisher's exact test and Pearson's chi-square test.

The probability model was applied to estimate the risk of tracheal aspiration.

A minimum significance level of 5% was considered for all tests.

3.12 RESEARCH ETHICS

This study was approved by the Ethics Committee, registration number CEP: 2099.2566/2009-11, on 12 March 2010. All the parents or guardians of the children who took part in the study signed the informed consent form (ICF) under registration number CEP: 2099.266/2009-11.

This study complements the previous study approved by the Research Ethics Committee of the Hospital de Clínicas, entitled "Comparative Analysis of Swallowing Sounds in Children with Cerebral Palsy and Normal Children assessed with Doppler Sonar", CAAE: 0278.0.208.000-09, with CEP registration: 2099.266/2009- 11, approved by this Committee on 12 March 2010.

3.13 RESEARCH MONITORING

The research was carried out taking into account protection measures, risk minimisation, confidentiality, the responsibility of the researcher and the institution, in accordance with the commitment signed with the Human Research Ethics Committee of the Hospital de Clínicas of the Federal University of Paraná when the project was submitted.

3.14 RESEARCH FUNDING

This research was supported by a scholarship provided by the Coordination for the Improvement of Higher Education Personnel (Capes).

CHAPTER 4

RESULTS

The study sample comprised 75 children diagnosed with CP (CP Group), complaining of dysphagia, aged between 0 and 15 years, 32 (42.7%) female and 43 (57.3%) male (Table 1). Of these, 72 (96.0%) had tetraplegia and 3 (4.0%) had hemiplegia. All the patients who took part in this study had a previous diagnosis of cerebral palsy and were referred for a VDF dynamic swallowing study due to complaints of dysphagia. The control group (Group C) was made up of 90 children with no swallowing complaints and no neuromotor alterations, aged between 2 and 15 years, 45 (50.0%) female and 45 (50.0%) male.

TABLE 1- DISTRIBUTION OF CEREBRAL PALSY AND CONTROL GROUPS ACCORDING TO SEX AND AGE

SEX AND AGE	PC group (n = 75)	Group C (n = 90)	P
Sex (M/F)	43/32	45/45	0,43
Age (years)			
0-5	46 (61,3%)	30 (33,3%)	0,001
6-10	14 (18,7%)	30 (33,3%)	
11-15	15 (20,0%)	30 (33,3%)	

SOURCE: The author (2107)

4.1 ANALYSING SWALLOWING USING VIDEOFLUOROSCOPY

Patients in Group PC underwent a clinical swallowing assessment and instrumental assessments that included VDF and Doppler sonar, while patients in Group C had acoustic swallowing data collected only by Doppler sonar.

According to the FDV, 50 children (67.0%) had mild dysphagia, 9 (12.0%) had moderate dysphagia and 16 (21.0%) had severe dysphagia, according to the classification of dysphagia severity by Ott et al. (1996).

Among the children with cerebral palsy, all (100.0%) showed alterations in the oral phase and 47 (62.7%) in the pharyngeal phase. Table 2 shows the alterations in the oral and pharyngeal phases observed in the FDV of the patients in the CP group.

TABLE 2- CHANGES IN THE ORAL AND PHARYNGEAL PHASES ACCORDING TO VIDEOFLUOROSCOPY IN THE GROUP OF PATIENTS WITH CEREBRAL PALSY

CHARACTERISTICS OBSERVED IN VIDEOFLUOROSCOPY	NO (n/%)	YES (n/%)
ORAL PHASE		
Ability to control food in the mouth	61 (81,3%)	14 (18,7%)

Difficulty sealing the lips	1 (1,3%)	74 (98,7%)
Early escape	11 (14,7%)	64 (85,3%)
Loss of oral reflexes	2 (2,7%)	73 (97,3%)
Altered movement of the anterior part and dorsum of the tongue	14 (18,7%)	61 (81,3%)
Reduced tongue control	1 (1,3%)	74 (98,7%)
Subsequent early escape	26 (34,7%)	49 (65,3%)
Clearance of oral contents	34 (45,3%)	41 (54,7%)
PHARINGEA PHASE		
Rhinopharyngeal drainage	68 (90,7%)	7 (9,3%)
Changes in laryngeal elevation and contraction	29 (38,7%)	46 (61,3%)
Tracheal penetration	47 (62,7%)	28 (37,3%)
Laryngotracheal aspiration	48 (64,0%)	27 (36%)
Silent suction	59 (78,7%)	16 (21,3%)
Presence and/or complaint of coughing during feeding	36 (48,0%)	39 (52,0%)
Presence of stasis in epiglottic vallecula and piriform recesses	36 (48,0%)	39 (52,0%)
Adequacy of the cricopharyngeus (upper oesophageal sphincter)	0 (0,0%)	75 (100,0%)

SOURCE: The author (2017).

Seventy children (93.3%) were being fed orally, 2 (2.7%) orally and by nasogastric tube, 1 (1.3%) exclusively via gastrostomy and 2 (2.7%) orally with supplementary feeding via gastrostomy.

4.2 ANALYSING SWALLOWING SOUNDS USING DOPPLER SONAR

Table 3 shows the acoustic profile of the swallowing sounds captured by the Doppler sonar during the swallowing of liquid, nectar and pudding in the children in the CP Group.

TABLE 3- ACOUSTIC PROFILE OF SWALLOWING SOUNDS CAPTURED BY DOPPLER SONAR IN LIQUID, NECTAR AND PUDDING FOOD CONSISTENCIES IN CHILDREN WITH CEREBRAL PALSY

VARIABLE AND CONSISTENCY	n	AVERAGE
LIQUID		
Initial Frequency 1 (FI1)	69	770,41 + 106,61
Peak Frequency 1 (FP1)	69	1025,78 + 95,20
Final Frequency 1 (FF1)	69	774,25 + 122,31
Initial Intensity 1 (II1)	69	65,97 + 8,36
Peak Intensity 1 (IP1)	69	86,28 + 7,51
Final Intensity 1 (IF1)	69	67,02 + 9,35
Time 1 (T1)	69	1,18 + 0,46
NECTAR (THIN PASTY)		
Initial Frequency 2 (FI2)	64	758,89 + 107,73
Peak Frequency 2 (FP2)	64	1028,56 + 106,57
Final Frequency 2 (FF2)	64	769,29 + 117,46
Initial Intensity 2 (II2)	64	65,06 + 8,60
Peak Intensity 2 (IP2)	64	86,40 + 8,46
Final Intensity 2 (IF2)	64	65,96 + 9,34
Time 2 (T2)	64	1,34 (0,61-4,27)
PUDDING (THICK PASTY)		
Initial Frequency 3 (FI3)	48	767,06 + 107,23
Peak Frequency 3 (FP3)	48	1032,66 + 89,93
Final Frequency 3 (FF3)	48	769,52 + 126,84
Initial Intensity 3 (II3)	48	65,60 + 8,64
Peak Intensity 3 (IP3)	48	86,73 + 7,07
Final Intensity 3 (IF3)	48	65,96 + 10,06
Time 3 (T3)	48	1,32 (0,56-2,65)

SOURCE: The author (2017)
NOTE: Frequencies measured in Hertz, Intensities measured in decibels, Times measured in seconds

4.2.1 Swallowing Sounds by Doppler Sonar in Children with Cerebral Palsy and a Control Group with Liquid Consistency

A comparative study of the acoustic parameters of swallowing sounds using Doppler sonar between the children in Group CP and Group C during the swallowing of liquid food revealed significant differences in FI1 - Initial Frequency, FP1 - Peak Frequency, II1 - Initial Intensity, IP1 - Peak Intensity and T1 - Swallowing Time.

During the synchronised VDF and Doppler sonar tests, 69 children swallowed liquid food. Table 4 shows the acoustic parameters of the swallowing sounds observed.

TABLE 4- CHARACTERISTICS OF THE ACOUSTIC PARAMETERS OF SWALLOWING SOUNDS OBSERVED BY DOPPLER SONAR WITH LIQUID CONSISTENCY

VARIABLE AND CONSISTENCY	PC GROUP (n = 69)	GROUP C (n = 90)	p
Initial Frequency 1 (FI1)	770,41±106,61	720,88±55,94	0.000[1]
Peak Frequency 1 (FP1)	1025,78±95,20	1099,93±15,87	0.000[1]
Initial Intensity 1 (II1)	65,97±8,36	62,18±4,43	0.000[1]
Peak Intensity 1 (IP1)	86,28±7,50	92,09±1,25	0.000[1]
Time 1 (T1)	1,18±0,46	0,97±0,23	0.000[2]

SOURCE: The author (2017)
NOTE:[1] Student's T-test,[2] Mann Whitney, Frequencies measured in Hertz, Intensities measured in decibels, Time measured in seconds.

4.2.2 Analysing swallowing sounds with Doppler sonar in fine pasty consistency (nectar)

During the VDF and Doppler sonar tests, 64 children swallowed food in the consistency of fine pasty (nectar). When comparing the acoustic parameters of swallowing sounds using Doppler sonar between the children in Group CP and Group C, a significant difference was observed in all the variables studied, namely: FI2 - Initial Frequency, FP2 - Peak Frequency, II2 - Initial Intensity, IP2 - Peak Intensity and T2 - Swallowing Time (Table 5).

TABLE 5- CHARACTERISTICS OF THE ACOUSTIC PARAMETERS OF SWALLOWING SOUNDS OBSERVED USING DOPPLER SONAR WITH A THIN PASTY CONSISTENCY - NECTAR

VARIABLE AND CONSISTENCY	PC GROUP (n = 64)	GROUP C (n = 90)	P
Initial Frequency 2 (FI2)	758,89±107,73	717,60±54,85	< 0,001[1]
Peak Frequency 2 (FP2)	1028,56±106,57	1085,96±26,56	< 0,001[1]
Initial Intensity 2 (II2)	65,06±8,60	61,91±4,33	< 0,001[1]
Peak Intensity 2 (IP2)	86,40±8,46	91,00±2,09	< 0,001[1]
Time 2 (T2)	1,34(0,61-4,27)	0,87+0,24	< 0,001[2]

SOURCE: The author (2017)
NOTE:[1] Student's t-test,[2] Main Whitney, Frequencies measured in Hertz, Intensities measured in decibels, Time measured in seconds.

4.2.3 Comparative analysis of swallowing sounds captured by Doppler sonar in a group of children with cerebral palsy

There was no significant difference when comparing the ratio of sound signals (frequency, intensity and time) in the three consistencies between males and females, age or consistencies used. However, there was a significant difference for the parameters of the acoustic signals according to the presence and absence of dysphagia, regardless of the severity of dysphagia, except for the initial intensity in the liquid (absence of dysphagia versus moderate dysphagia) and fine pasty (absence of dysphagia versus mild dysphagia) consistencies (Table 6).

TABLE 6- CHARACTERISTICS OF THE ACOUSTIC PARAMETERS OF SWALLOWING IN CHILDREN WITH AND WITHOUT CEREBRAL PALSY AND THE SEVERITY OF DYSPHAGIA

VARIABLE E CONSISTENCY	NORMAL DEGLUTATION (n=90)	MILD DYSPHAGIA (n=45)	MODERATE dysphagia (n=9)	Severe dysphagia (n=15)	P1	p2	p3	P4
FI 1 (Hz)	720,88+55,94	776,83+118,29	746,82+61,34	765,30+92,52	0,001[1]	0,001[1]	0,001[1]	p>0,05[1]
FP 1 (Hz)	1099,93+15,87	1028,76+104,04	1010,16+96,61	1026,23+66,92	0,001[1]	0,001[1]	0,001[1]	p > 0,05[1]
II 1 (dB)	62,18+4,43	66,43+9,27	64,22+4,84	68,20+5,45	0,001[1]	0,17[1]	0,001[1]	p > 0,05[1]
IP 1 (dB)	92,09+1,25	86,47+8,2	85,34+7,71	89,12+3,89	0,001[1]	0,001[1]	0,001[1]	p > 0,05[1]
T 1 (s)	0,95(0,53-1,92)	1,21(0,42-2,4)	1,27(0,71-1,77)	0,99(0,40-1,97)	0,008[2]	0,009[2]	0,23[2]	p>0,05[2]
FI 2 (Hz)	717,60+54,85	743,62+118,92	778,69+82,42	797,22+69,16	0,008[1]	0,004[1]	0,001[1]	p > 0,05[1]
FP 2 (Hz)	1085,96+26,56	1013,89+123,41	1052,63+50,77	1062,25+49,29	0,001[1]	0,002[1]	0,009[1]	p > 0,05[1]
II 2 (dB)	61,91+4,33	63,80+9,50	66,74+6,50	68,20+5,45	0,11[1]	0,004[1]	0,001[1]	p > 0,05[1]
IP 2 (dB)	91,00+2,09	85,22+9,79	88,36+4,00	89,12+3,89	0,001[1]	0,002[1]	0,009[1]	p>0,05[1]
T 2 (s)	0,87(0,42-1,72)	1,38(0,61-4,2)	1,10(0,69-1,95)	1,02(0,69-1,85)	0,001[2]	0,004[2]	0,001[2]	p >0,05[2]

SOURCE: The author (2017).
NOTE:[1] Student's t-test [2] Mann-Whitney test p1= comparison between absence of dysphagia and mild dysphagia; p2= comparison between absence of dysphagia and moderate dysphagia, p3= comparison between absence of dysphagia and severe dysphagia, p4= comparison between mild, moderate and severe dysphagia. FI1= initial liquid frequency, FP1= peak liquid frequency, II1= initial liquid intensity, IP1= peak liquid intensity, T1= liquid time, FI2= initial nectar frequency, FP2= peak nectar frequency, II2= initial nectar intensity, IP2= peak nectar intensity, T2= nectar time.

There was no association between the severity of dysphagia and the age of the children with cerebral palsy.When analysing the sound signals (frequency, intensity and time) of the children with cerebral palsy according to the presence or absence of aspiration, there was no significant difference (Table

7), except for the consistency of thick pasty, where the time was significantly longer (p=0.04) in the children with cerebral palsy and aspiration.

TABLE 7- ACOUSTIC PARAMETERS OF SWALLOWING SOUNDS IN CHILDREN WITH CEREBRAL PALSY WITH AND WITHOUT ASPIRATION

VARIABLE AND CONSISTENCY	n	NO ASPIRATION Mean + SD/Median	n	WITH ASPIRATION Mean + SD/Median	P
Initial Frequency 1 (FI1)	43	775,24±120,24	26	762,40±80,72	0,63[1]
Peak Frequency 1 (FP1)	43	1023,56±105,88	26	1029,44±76,11	0,80[1]
Initial Intensity 1 (II1)	43	66,29±9,42	26	65,44±6,39	0,68[1]
Peak Intensity 1 (IP1)	43	86,06±8,35	26	86,65±6,01	0,75[1]
Time 1 (T1)	43	1,23(0,42-2,38)	26	1,11(0,40-2,47)	0,50[2]
Initial Frequency 2 (FI2)	41	744,44±121,31	23	762,40±80,72	0,15[1]
Peak Frequency 2 (FP2)	41	1013,59±125,15	23	1029,44±76,11	0,13[1]
Initial Intensity 2 (II2)	41	63,99±9,57	23	66,95±6,28	0,18[1]
Peak Intensity 2 (IP2)	41	85,26±9,88	23	88,44±4,55	0,15[1]
Time 2 (T2)	41	1,38(0,61-4,27)	23	1,06(0,63-2,04)	0,13[2]
Initial Frequency 3 (FI3)	27	756,51±123,55	21	780,62±82,65	0,44[1]
Peak Frequency 3 (FP3)	27	1024,26±92,70	21	1043,47±87,27	0,46[1]
Initial Intensity 3 (II3)	27	64,60±10,00	21	66,89±6,52	0,36[1]
Peak Intensity 3 (IP3)	27	86,05±7,27	21	87,62±6,88	0,45[1]
Time 3 (T3)	27	1,24(0,56-2,65)	21	1,49(0,88-2,51)	0,04[2]

SOURCE: The author (2017)
NOTE:[1] Student's t-test,[2] Mann Whitney. Measures for initial and peak frequencies: Hz= Hertz, measures for initial and peak intensity: dB=decibels, measure for time: s= seconds

None of the acoustic parameters observed by Doppler sonar were predictive of tracheal aspiration, either by analysing the sensitivity and specificity indices by constructing Roc curves or by analysing the multivariate logistic regression model (p > 0.05) (Table 8).

TABLE 8- MULTIVARIATE LOGISTIC REGRESSION OF ACOUSTIC PARAMETERS OF SWALLOWING SOUNDS OF CHILDREN WITH CEREBRAL PALSY WHO HAD ASPIRATION (VDF) CAPTURED BY DOPPLER SONAR

VARIABLE AND CONSISTENCY	OR	95% CI
LIQUID		
Initial Frequency 1 (FI1)	0,99	0,98 - 1,00
Peak Frequency 1 (FP1)	0,99	0,98 - 1,00
Initial Intensity 1 (II1)	0,94	0,83 - 1,06
Peak Intensity 1 (IP1)	0,99	0,87 - 1,12
NECTAR (THIN PASTY)		
Initial Frequency 2 (FI2)	1,00	0,99 - 1,01
Peak Frequency 2 (FP2)	1,00	0,99 - 1,01
Initial Intensity 2 (II2)	1,08	0,95 - 1,22
Peak Intensity 2 (IP2)	1,07	0,94 - 1,23
PUDDING (THICK PASTY)		
Initial Frequency 3 (FI3)	1,00	0,99 - 1,01
Peak Frequency 3 (FP3)	0,99	0,99 - 1,00
Initial Intensity 3 (II3)	1,01	0,88 - 1,16
Peak Intensity 3 (IP3)	0,99	0,89 - 1,10

SOURCE: The author (2017)
NOTE: Multivariate logistic regression OR = Odds Ratio CI = Confidence Interval

In the univariate logistic regression, fine pasty time was the only variable in the acoustic parameter of swallowing sounds captured by Doppler sonar that could suggest a risk of tracheal aspiration

(Graph 1) for aspiration, as can be seen in Graph 1.

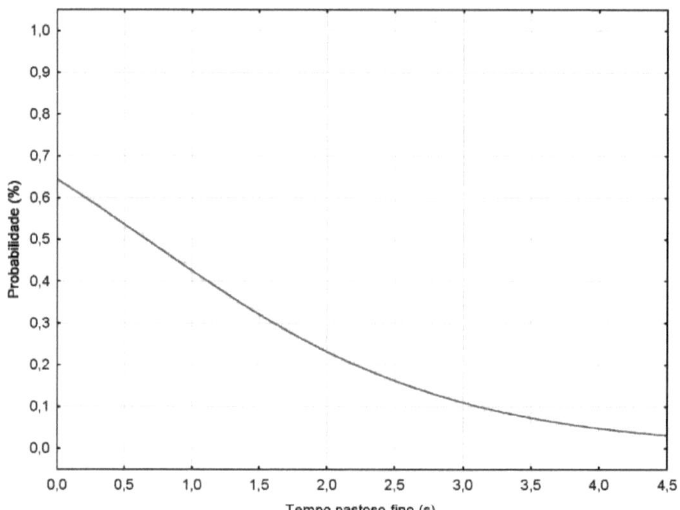

GRAPH 1 - PROBABILITY OF TRACHEAL ASPIRATION ACCORDING TO FINE PASTY TIME
SOURCE: The author (2017)
NOTE: Logistic Regression - Probability Model (p = 0.08)

There was no significant difference in the acoustic parameters of swallowing between children who had non-silent aspiration on VDF (10 children) and silent aspiration (16 children) (p > 0.05).

Even considering the paired analysis by sex and age with 49 children in each group, the results were similar (p > 0.05).

CHAPTER 5

DISCUSSION

Based on studies of swallowing sounds already carried out in patients without dysphagia, the sound variables of more adequate swallowing have a higher frequency and intensity, with a shorter time, which indicates better performance in the swallowing process (SANTOS; MACEDO FILHO, 2006; CAGLIARI et al., 2009; SPADOTTO, 2010; LAGOS et al., 2013; SORIA; SILVA; FURKIM, 2016).

In this study, the swallowing sounds observed during the feeding of liquid and pasty foods (nectar), captured by Doppler sonar in children with cerebral palsy and the control group, carried out synchronously with the assessment of swallowing using videofluoroscopy, made it possible to draw a different sound curve in children with dysphagia.

In this way, the differences in sound variables found in this study with children with cerebral palsy may suggest the presence of pharyngeal alterations during sound capture of swallowing with Doppler sonar. There are no additional studies evaluating swallowing sounds with Doppler sonar in children with dysphagia (LAGARDE; KAMALSKI; ENGEL- HOEK, 2016).

Some other published studies analyse swallowing sounds using Doppler sonar, Abdulmassih et al. (2013) analysed the variables of frequency, time and intensity for swallowing sounds, comparing the results obtained between two groups of 30 adults, one with and one without dominant spinocerebellar ataxia. They observed significant differences in sound signal wave patterns during swallowing, similar to those found in cerebral palsy patients in the present study. These authors also observed higher Initial Frequency (IF) and Initial Intensity (II), as well as lower Peak Frequency (PF) and Peak Intensity (PI) in their patients with spinocerebellar ataxia, the results being attributed to motor dysfunction. Sória et al. (2016) compared the acoustic parameters of swallowing between adults with no complaints of dysphagia at different ages, correlating swallowing and ageing, analysing 75 elderly adults and 72 young adults, obtaining results that showed a reduction in muscle movement in elderly adults with a reduction in laryngeal elevation (FI and II) and an increase in swallowing time (T) in elderly adults.

In this study of children with cerebral palsy, the mean initial frequency (IF) and initial intensity (IF), which represent laryngeal elevation and the start of the pharyngeal phase of swallowing, were higher among children with cerebral palsy compared to the control group, in both consistencies studied. These data suggest altered muscle strength and altered mobility of laryngeal elevation and contraction, with a probable higher movement to protect the larynx in order to avoid aspiration of food.

The mean peak frequency (PF) and peak intensity (PI), which indicate cricopharyngeal opening, were lower in the group of children with CP compared to the control group, in both consistencies studied, results that may be related to the motor disability.

The time medians (T), which indicate the duration from the beginning to the end of the acoustic signal captured, showed an increase in swallowing time in the children in the study group, which corroborates that observed in other studies, such as Vivone et al. (2007); Lustre, Freire and Silvério (2013); both of which used a stopwatch during a clinical assessment to analyse oropharyngeal swallowing time in children with CP; and Tamanini (2013), who used a microphone and VDF.

The swallowing time assessed in this study refers to the sound captured from the pharyngeal phase, with laryngeal elevation until the structures return to their resting position, and is not directly related to swallowing time from the oral phase.

Although the results may be limited by the presence of tracheal aspiration in only 27 children, when the parameters of the frequency and intensity sound signals of children with CP with and without aspiration were studied, no significant difference was observed, corroborating the results found by Tamanini (2013). The duration of the pharyngeal phase during swallowing with a thick pasty consistency was significantly longer in patients with CP and aspiration when compared to those with CP without aspiration. In the present study, the fine pasty time suggested a risk for aspiration that was inversely proportional to time. These data of a longer time for the thick pasty consistency and a shorter time for the thin pasty consistency related to the risk of aspiration suggest that altered pharyngeal mobility in cerebral palsy and the severity of dysphagia are important factors for the risk of aspiration, i.e. in severe dysphagia the thin pasty food goes down by gravity (fast) and the thick pasty food, which requires propulsive force and mobility, with the motor alteration, has its time prolonged; which in both cases favours aspiration.

There was no difference in sound signals (frequency, intensity and time) according to gender, which shows that in this pathology, the sequelae of oropharyngeal dysphagia are similar for boys and girls, in line with the studies by Pfeifer et al. (2009), Newmann et al. (2001), Weir et al. (2011) and Lynch et al. (2008), with different study populations.

There was no significant difference in the sound signals (frequency, intensity and time) between the three food consistencies studied: liquid, fine pasty and coarse pasty. The sound signals picked up by Doppler sonar did not show any better indication of oropharyngeal perception and control when comparing the different types of food consistency, corroborating the study carried out by Curado, Garcia and Di Francesco (2005) in children with CP, Lee et al.

(2016) through FDV in normal adults with different consistencies. There was also no improvement in sound patterns for the fine pasty consistency (nectar), as seen in the studies by Jestrovic et al. (2013) using an accelerometer in adults with normal swallowing, which shows that in this study with children with CP, the severity of dysphagia overrides an improvement in perception and consequent better motor control of swallowing with different types of food consistency. Contrary to the studies carried out by Lustre, Freire and Silvério (2013), with children with CP, through clinical assessment and a chronometer, they observed differences in food consistencies and swallowing. Ruark, Mills and Muenchen (2003) studied healthy adults and children using electromyography and cervical auscultation, Aurélio, Genaro and Macedo-Filho (2002) studied children with and without CP using clinical assessment and a chronometer, and found the same results.

This study also found no significant difference in sound signals (frequency, intensity and time) according to the age groups of children with CP, which shows that the sequelae of dysphagia are not related to differences in age, in agreement with the study by Weir et al. (2011). These authors found that age was not associated with silent or non-silent aspiration in children with oropharyngeal dysphagia assessed by VDF. Cagliari et al. (2009), however, analysed the swallowing sounds of 90 children between the ages of 2 and 15 without complaints of dysphagia, describing age-related differences, finding lower frequency and intensity of the sound signals generated during swallowing in the younger group, which increased with age, probably due to the difference in the size of the larynx.

During the instrumental phonoaudiological assessment using the dynamic swallowing study by VDF, the children with CP showed various oral and pharyngeal alterations, with the presence of aspiration. These data confirm the high prevalence of oropharyngeal dysphagia in patients with CP, as described by Mirrett et al. (1994), Rogers et al. (1994), Furkim, Behlau; Weckx (2003), Curado; Garcia; Di Francesco (2005), Marrara et al. (2008), Kim et al. (2013), Lustre; Freire; Silvério (2013), Engel-Hock et al. (2014), Benfer et al. (2014), Benfer et al. (2015), Suet al. (2016).

The results found in this study suggest that the swallowing process in patients with CP, as well as being slower due to oropharyngeal dysphagia, results from difficulties in controlling muscle tone and the mobility of the muscle structures involved in the process.

Further studies are needed to standardise the curves of the acoustic signals of swallowing and to simultaneously analyse the sound with the image of the swallowing process using specific software. A non-invasive, quick and accessible way of assessing children with CP, especially to determine the risk of prandial aspiration, could substantially improve their quality of life.

CHAPTER 6

CONCLUSION

a) The mean Initial Frequency (IF) and Initial Intensity (II) for the two consistencies studied and the median time (T) were higher among the children with cerebral palsy, while the mean Peak Frequency (PF) and Peak Intensity (PI) were lower.

b) Prolonged time in the thick pasty consistency and reduced time in the thin pasty consistency were the acoustic parameters found that may suggest a risk of aspiration.

FINAL CONSIDERATIONS

The use of Doppler sonar equipment to capture swallowing sounds has proved to be a viable and auxiliary resource for analysing swallowing sounds, as it provides numerical and measurable data as a screening method.

Doppler sonar can be useful as a screening method during speech therapy care for children with cerebral palsy. Although it is promising in aiding the diagnosis and follow-up of patients with dysphagia, videofluoroscopy and nasofibrolaryngoscopy remain the gold standard methods for accurate diagnosis.

REFERENCES

ABDULMASSIH, E. M.S.; TEIVE, H. A. G.; SANTOS, R. S.The evaluation of swallowing in patients with spinocerebellar ataxia and oropharyngeal dysphagia: A comparison study of videofluoroscopy and sonar Doppler. Intl Arch Otorhinolaryngol, n.17, p.66-73, 2013.

ADA. National Dysphagia Diet: Standardisation for Optimal Care. American Dietetic Association, 2002, p. 47. Chicago.

ARAÚJO, L. A.; SILVA, L. R.; MENDES, F. A. A. Digestive tract neural control and gastrointestinal disorders in cerebral palsy. J Pediatr, n.88, v.6, p.455-464, 2012.

ARVEDSON, J. C. Feeding children with cerebral palsy and swallowing difficulties. EJCN, n.67, p.9-12, 2013.

ARVEDSON, J.; ROGERS, B.; BUCK.G.; SMART.P.; MSALL, M. Silent aspiration prominent in children with dysphagia. Int. J. Pediatr. Otorhinolaryngol., n.28, p.173-181, 1994.

ASHA. Guidelines for Speech-Language Pathologists Performing Videofluoroscopic Swallowing Studies. ASHA Special Interest Division 13, Swallowing and Swallowing Disorders (Dysphagia). DIKEMAN, K.; GREEN, J.; HISS, S.; INMAN, A.; KELCHNER, L.; LAZARUS, C.; MILLER, C. 2004, access : http://www.asha.org/policy/GL2004-00050/#sec1.2

AURELIO, S. R.; GENARO, K. F.; MACEDO-FILHO, E. D. F. Comparative analysis of swallowing patterns in children with cerebral palsy and normal children. Rev. Bras. Otorrinol, v.68, n. 2, 167-173, 2002.

BAE, S. O.; GANG, P. L.; SEO, H. G.; BYUNG-MO, O.; TAI, R. H. Clinical characteristics associated with aspiration or penetration in children with swallowing problem. Ann Rehabil Med, n.38, v.6, p.734-741, 2014.

BAX, M.; GOLDSTEIM, M.; ROSENBAUM, P.; LEVINTON, A.; PANETH, N. Proposed definition and classification of cerebral palsy. Dev Med Child Neurol, v.47, p.571-576, 2005.

BEHLAU & MICHALIS. VoxMetria - Software for Analysing Voice and Vocal Quality. CTS Informática, 2003.

BENFER, K. A.; WEIR, K. A.; BELL, K. L.; WARE, R. S.; DAVIES, P. S. W.; BOYD, R. N. Clinical signs suggestive of pharyngeal dysphagia in preschool children with cerebral palsy. Research in Developmental Disabilities, n.38, p.192-201, 2015.

BENFER, K. A.; WEIR, K. A.; BELL, K. L.; WARE, R. S.; DAVIES, P. S. W.; BOYD, R. N. Oropharyngeal dysphagia in preschool children with cerebral palsy: oral phase impairments. Research in Developmental Disabilities, n. 35, p. 3469-3481, 2014.

BENFER, K. A.; WEIR, K. A.; BELL, K. L.; WARE, R. S.; DAVIES, P. S. W.; BOYD, R. N. The Eating and Drinking Ability the Classification System in a population-based sample of preschool children with cerebral palsy. Research in Developmental Disabilities, n.59, p.647-654, 2017.

BOBATH, K. Motor paralysis in patients with cerebral palsy. São Paulo, 2ed.Manole, 1984.

BOLZAN, G. P.; CHRISTMANN, M. K.; BERWIG, L. C.; COSTA, C. C.; ROCHA, R. M. Contribution of cervical auscultation to the clinical evaluation of oropharyngeal dysphagia. Rev CEFAC, n.15, v.2, p.455-465, 2013.

BORR, C.; HIELSHER-FASTABEND, M.; PHIL, D. R.; LUCKING, A. Reliability and validity of cervical auscultation. Dysphagia, n.22, p.225-234, 2007.

BRASILEIRO, I. C.; MOREIRA, T. M. M.; JORGE, M. S. B.; QUEIROZ, M. V. O.; MONT ÁLVERNE, D. G. B. Activities and participation of children with Cerebral Palsy according to the International Classification of Functioning, Disability and Health. Rev Bras Enferm, n. 62, p. 503-511, 2009.

CAGLIARI, C. F.; JURKIEWICZ, A. L.; SANTOS, R. S.; MARQUES, J. M.Doppler sonar analysis of swallowing sounds in normal paediatric individuals. Braz J Otorhinolaryngol, n.75, p.706-715, 2009.

CANS, C. Surveillance of cerebral palsy in Europe: a collaboration of cerebral palsy surveys and registers. Dev Med Child Neurol, n.42, p.816-824, 2000.

CARDOSO, M. C. A. F.; FONTOURA, E. G. Value of cervical auscultation in patients with neurogenic dysphagia. Intl. Arch. Otorhinolaryngol, n.13, v.4, p.431-439, 2009.

CARVALHO, A. P. C.; CHIARI, B. M.; GOLÇALVES,M. .IR. Impact of an educational programme on the diet of neuropathic children. CoDAS, n.25, v.5, p.413-421, 2013.

CHAGAS, P. S. C.; DEFILIPO, E. C.; LEMOS, R. A.; MANCINI, M. C.; FRÔNIO, J. S.; CARVALHO, R. M. Classification of motor function and functional performance in children with cerebral palsy. Rev Bras Fisioter, n.12, p.409- 416, 2008.

CICHERO, J. A. Y.; MURDOCH, B. E. The physiologic cause of swallowing sounds: answers from heart sounds and vocal tract acoustics. Dysphagia, n.13, p.39-52, 1998.

COLA, P. C.; GATTO, A. R.; SILVA, R. G.; SCHELP, A. O.; HENRY, M. A. C. A. Rehabilitation in neurogenic oropharyngeal dysphagia: sour taste and cold temperature. Rev CEFAC, n.10, v.2, p.200-205, 2008.

CURADO, A. D. F.; GARCIA, R. S. P.; DI FRANCESCO, R. C. Investigation of silent aspiration in patients with spastic tetraparetic cerebral palsy through videofluoroscopic examination. Rev CEFAC, n.7, p. 188-197, 2005.

DE MATTEO, C.; MATOVICH, D.; HJARTASON, A. Comparison of clinical and videofluoroscopic evaluation of children with feeding and swallowing difficulties. Dev Med Child Neurol, n.47, p.149-157, 2005.

EICHER, P. P. S.; MANO, C. J.; FOX, C. A.; KERWIN, M. E. Impact of cervical auscultation on accuracy of clinical evaluation in predicting penetration/aspiration in a paediatric population. Minute-Second workshop on cervical auscultation. Mc Lean, Virginia, October 13, 1994. p. 28-32.

ENGEL-KOEK, L.; ERASMUS, C. E.; HULST, K. C. M.; ARVEDSON, J. C.; GROOT, I. J. M.; SWART, B. J. M. Children with central and peripheral neurologic disorders have distinguishable patterns of dysphagia on videofluoroscopic swallow study. Journal of Child Neurology, n.29, v.5, p.646-653, 2014.

FRAKKING, T. T.; CHANG, A. B.; O'GRADY, K. A. F.; WALKER-SMITH, K.; WEIR, K. A. Cervical auscultation in the diagnosis of oropharyngeal aspiration in children: a study protocol for a randomised controlled trial. Trials, n. 14, p. 377, 2013.

FUNAYAMA, C. A. R.; MOURA-RIBEIRO, M. V. L.; GONÇALVES, A. L. Hypoxic-ischaemic encephalopathy in term newborns. Arq Neuropsiquiatr, n.55, v.4, p.771-779, 1997.

FURKIM, A. M.; BEHLAU, M.; WECKX, L. L. M. Clinical and videofluoroscopic evaluation of swallowing in children with cerebral palsy. Arq Neuropsiquiatr, n.61, v.3, p.611-616, 2003.

FURKIM, A. M.; DUARTE, S. T.; SACCA, A. F. B.; SÓRIA, F. S. The use of cervical auscultation in inferring tracheal aspiration in children with cerebral palsy. Rev CEFAC, n.11, v.4, p.624-629, 2009.

FURKIM, A. M.; SACCO, A. B. F. Effectiveness of speech therapy in neurogenic dysphagia using the functional oral intake scale (FOIS) as a marker. Rev CEFAC, n.10, v.4, p.503-512, 2008.

GONÇALVES, M. I. R.; VIDIGAL, M. L. N. In: FURKIM, A. M.; SANTINI, C. S. Dysfagias Orofaríngeas, Pró-Fono, p.189-201, 1999.

GRIGS, C. A.; JONES, P. M.; LEE, R. E. Videofluoroscopic investigation of feeding disorders in children with multiple handicap. Dev Med Child Neurol, n.131, p.303-308, 1989.

GROHER, M. E. In: FURKIM, A. M.; SANTINI, C. S. Oropharyngeal Dysphagia, Pró-Fono, p. 97-107, 1999.

HAMLET, S. L.; NELSON, R. J.; PATTERSON, R. L. Interpreting the sounds of swallowing; fluid flow through the cricopharyngeus. Ann Otol Rhinol Laryngol, n.99, p.749-752, 1990.

HAMLET, S. L.; PATTERSON, R. L.; FLEMING, S. M.; JONES, L. A. Sounds of Swallowing following total laryngectomy. Dysphagia, n.7, p.160-165, 1992.

HAMMOUDI, K.; BOIRON, M.; HERNANDEZ, N.; BOBILLIER, C.; MORINIE'RE, S. Acoustic study of pharyngeal swallowing as a function of the volume and consistency of the bolus. Dysphagia, n. 29, p. 468-474, 2014.

HIDECKER, M. J. C.; PANETH, N.; ROSENBAUM, P.L.; KENT, R.D.; LILIE, J.; EULENBERG, J. B.; CHESTER JR, K.; JOHNSON, B.; MICHALSEN, L.; EVATT, M.; TAYLOR, K. Developing and validating the Communication Function Classification System for individuals with cerebral palsy. Dev Med Child Neurol, n. 53, v. 8, p. 704-710, 2011.

HIRATA, G. C.; SANTOS, R. S. Rehabilitation of oropharyngeal dysphagia in children with cerebral palsy: a systematic review of the phonoaudiological approach. Int Arch Otorhinolaryngol, n.16, v.3, p.396-399, 2012.

JAFFER, N. M.; WING-FAI, A. F.; STEELE, C. M. Fluoroscopic evaluation of oro-pharyngeal dysphagia: anatomy, technique, and common etiologies. AJR Am J Roentegenol, n. 204, v. 1, p. 49-58, 2015.

JESTROVI, I.; DUDIK, J. M.; LUAN, B.; COYLE, J. L.; SEJDI, E. The effects of increased fluid viscosity on swallowing sounds in healthy adults. BioMedical Engineering OnLine,n.12, p.90, 2013.

KAHRILAS, P. J.; SHEZLANG, L.; RADEMAKER, A. W.; LOGEMANN, J. A. Impaired Deglutitive airway protection: a videofluoroscopic analysis of severity and mechanism. Gastroenterology, n.113, v.5, p.1457-1464, 1997.

KIM, J. S.; HAM, Z. A.; SONG, D. H.; OH, H. M. Characteristics of dysphagia in children with cerebral palsy related to Gross Motor Function. Am J Phys Med Rehabil, n.92, p. 912-919, 2013.

KRIGGER, K. W. Cerebral palsy: an overview. Am Fam Physician, n.73, v.1, p.91-100, 2006.

LAGARDE, M. L. J.; KAMALSKI, D. M. A.; ENGEL-HOEK, L. V. The reliability and validity of cervical auscultation in the diagnosis of dysphagia: a systematic review. Clinical Rehabilitation, n.30, v.2, p.199-207, 2016.

LAGOS, H. N. C.; SANTOS, R. S.; ABDULMASSIH, E. M. S.; GALLINEA, L. F.; LANGONE, M. Characterisation of swallowing sounds with the use of sonar Doppler in full-term and preterm newborns. Intl Arch Otorhinolaryngol, n.17, p.383-386, 2013.

LAGOS-GUIMARÃES, H. N. C.; TEIVE, H. A. G.; CELLI, A.; SANTOS, R. S.; ABDULMASSIH, E. M. S.; HIRATA, G. C.; GALLINEA, L. F. Aspiration pneumonia in children with cerebral palsy after videofluoroscopic swallowing study. Intl Arch Otorhinolaryngol, n.20, p. 132-137, 2016.

LESLIE, P.; DRINNAN, M. J.; ZAMMIT-MAEMPEL, I.; COYLE, J. L.; FORD, G. A.; WILSON, J. A. Cervical auscultation synchronised with images from endoscopy swallow evaluations. Dysphagia, n.22, p.290-298, 2007.

LOGEMAN, J. A. Swallowing disorders. Best Pract Res Cl Ga, n.21, p.563- 573, 2007.

LUSTRE, N. S.; FREIRE, T. R. B.; SILVERIO, C. C. Oral transit time measurements in children with cerebral palsy of different motor levels and their relationship with the degree of severity for dysphagia. ACR, n.18, p.155-161, 2013.

LYNCH, C. S.; CHAMMAS, M. C.; MANSUR, L. L.; CERRI, G. G. Ultrasound biomechanics of swallowing: preliminary study. Radiol Bras, n.41, v.4, p.241-244, 2008.

MANRIQUE, D.; MELO, E. C. M.; BUHLER, R. B. Nasofibrolaryngoscopic changes in swallowing in chronic non-progressive encephalopathy. J Pediat, n. 78, p. 67-70, 2002.

MARCHESAN, I. Q. Normal swallowing. In: FURKIM, A. M.; SANTINI, C. S. Oropharyngeal Dysphagia, Pró-Fono, p.3-18, 1999.

MARRARA, J. L.; DUCA, A. P.; DANTAS, R. O.; TRAWITZKI, L. V. V.; LIMA, R. A. C.; PEREIRA, J. C. Swallowing in children with neurological disorders: clinical and videofluoroscopic evaluation. Pró-Fono,n.20, v.4, p.231-236, 2008.

MCKAIG, T. N. Cervical and thoracic auscultation. In: FURKIM, A. M.; SANTINI, C. S. Oropharyngeal Dysphagia, Pró-Fono, p. 171-187, 1999.

MCKAIG, N.; STROUD, A. The comparison of swallowing sounds with simultaneously recorded fluoroscopic imaging. Dysphagia, n.12, p.30, 1997.

MINEAR, W.L. Special article: A classification of cerebral palsy. Paediatrics, n.18, p.841-852,1956.

MORINIÈRE, S.; BEUTTER, P.; BOIRON, M. Sound Component Duration of Healthy Human Pharyngoesophageal Swallowing: A Gender Comparison Study. Dysphagia, n. 21, p.175-182, 2006.

MORINIÈRE, S.; BOIRON, M.; ALISON, D.; MAKRIS, P.; BEUTTER, P. Origin of the sound components during pharyngeal swallowing in normal subjects. Dysphagia, n.23, p.267-273, 2008.

MORRIS, C. The definition and classification of cerebral palsy, historical perspective. Dev Med Child Neurol, n.109, p.3-7, 2007.

NEWMANN, L. A.; KECKLEY, C.; PETERSEN, M. C.; HAMMER, A. Swallowing function and medical diagnosis in infants suspected of dysphagia. PEDIATRICS, n.108, v.6, p. 106-108, 2001.

OTT, D. J.; HODGE, R. G.; PIKNA, L. A.; CHEN, M. Y.; GELFAND, D. W. Modified barium swallow: clinical and radiographic correlation and relation to feeding recommendations. Dysphagia, n.11, p.187-190, 1996.

PADOVANI, A. R.; MORAES, D. P.; MANGILI, L. D.; ANDRADE, C. R. F. Protocolo fonoaudiológico de avaliação de risco para dysfagia (PARD) Rev Soc Bras Fonoaudiol, n.12, v.3, p.199-205, 2007.

PATATAS, O. H. G.; GONÇALVES, M. I. R.; CHIARI, B. M.; GIELOW, I. Duration parameters of acoustic signals of swallowing in individuals without complaints. Rev Soc Bras Fonoaudiol, n. 16, v.3, p.282-290, 2011.

PAULA, A.; BOTELHO, I.;SILVA, A. A.; REZENDE, J. M. M.; FARIAS, C.; MENDES, L.

Evaluation of paediatric dysphagia through videoendoscopy of swallowing. Rev Bras Otorrinolaringol, n.68, p.91-96, 2002.

PENNY, L. M.; RISKI, J. E.; GLASCOTTJ, JOHNSON, V. Videofluoroscopic assessment of dysphagia in children with severe spastic cerebral palsy. Dysphagia, n. 9, p. 174-179, 1994.

PFEIFER, L. I.; SILVA, D. B. R.; FUNAYAMA, C. A. R.; SANTOS, J. L. Classification of cerebral palsy, association between gender, ager, motor type, topography and gross motor function. Arq Neuropsiquiatr, n. 67, v. 4, p.1057- 1061, 2009.

PINTO, A. R.; COLA, P. C.; CARVALHO, L. R.; MOTONAGA, S. M.; SILVA, R. G. Oral intake and degree of impairment in pre- and post-phonotherapy neurogenic oropharyngeal dysphagia. Rev Neurocienc, n.21, v.4, p. 531-536, 2013.

QUINTELLA, T.; SILVA, A. A.; BOTELHO, M. I. M. R.. In: FURKIM, A. M.; SANTINI, C. S. Oropharyngeal dysphagia, Pró-Fono, p.61-96, 1999.

RIBEIRO, M. O.; RAHAL, R. O.; KOKANJ, A. S.; BITTAR, D. P. The use of Kinesio elastic bandage in the control of sialorrhoea in children with cerebral palsy. ACTA FISIATR, n.16, v.4, p.168-172, 2009.

ROGERS, B.; ARVEDSON, J.; BUCK, G.; SMART, P.; MSALL, M. Characteristcs of dysphagia in children of cerebral palsy. Dysphagia, n. 9, p.69-73, 1994.

ROTTA, N. T. Cerebral palsy, new therapeutic perspectives. J Pediat, n.78, p.48-54, 2002.

RUAK, J. L.; MILLS, C. E.; NUENCHEN, R. A. Effects of bolus volume and consistency on multiple swallow behaviour in children and adults. Journal of Medical Speech-Language Pathology, n. 11, v. 4, p. 213, 2003.

SANKAR, C.; MUNDIKUR, N. Cerebral palsy - Definition, classification, etiology and early diagnosis. Indian J Pediatr, n.72, v.10, p.865-868, 2005.

SANTINI, C. S. Neurogenic dysphagia. In: Furkim AM &Santini CS. Oropharyngeal dysphagia, Pró-Fono, p.19-34, 1999.

SANTOS, R. J. F. Studies of swallowing by videofluoroscopy: the role of the speech therapist. Monograph (Specialisation in Speech Therapy) - Portuguese Catholic University, Lisbon, p. 49, 2013.

SANTOS, R. S.; MACEDO FILHO, E. D. Sonar Doppler as an instrument of deglutition evaluation. Intl Arch Otorhinolaryngology, n.10, p.182-191, 2006.

SILVA, C. S. Evaluation of sucking/swallowing/breathing through digital cervical auscultation in preterm and term newborns. Dissertation (Master's in Child and Adolescent Health) - Federal University of Rio Grande do Sul, Porto Alegre, p. 103, 2013.

SILVEIRA, R. C.; PROCIANOY, RS. Cerebral ischaemic lesions in very low birth weight preterm infants. J Pediatr, n.81, v.1, p.23-32, 2005.

SILVÉRIO, C. C.; HENRIQUE, C. S. Indicators of the evolution of patients with cerebral palsy and oropharyngeal dysphagia after therapeutic intervention. Rev Soc Bras Fonoaudiol, n.14, v.3, p.381-386, 2009.

SÓRIA, F. S.; SILVA, R. G.; FURKIM, A. M. Acoustic analysis of oropharyngeal swallowing using sonar doppler. Braz J Otorhinolaryngol, n.82, p.39-46, 2016.

SPADOTTO, A. A.; GATTO, A. R.; COLA, P. C.; MONTAGNOLI, A. N.; SCHELP, A. O.; SILVA, R. G.; YAMASHITA, S.; PEREIRA, J. C.; HENRY, M. A. C. A. Software for quantitative analysis of swallowing. Radiol Bras, n.41, v.1, p.25-28, 2008.

SPADOTTO, A. A.; GATTO, A. R.; COLA, P. C.; SILVA, R. G.; SCHELP, A. O.; SILVA, R. G.; DOMENIS, D. R.; DANTAS, R. O. Components of the acoustic signal of swallowing: preliminary study. J Soc Bras Fonoaudiol,n.24, v.3, p.218-222, 2012.

SU, C. L.; CHEN, S. L.; TSAI, S. W.; TSENG, F. E.; CHANG, S. C.; HUANG, Y. H.; LIN, Y. H. Efficacy of predicting videofluoroscopic results in dysphagic patients with severe cerebral palsy using de Mann assesment of swallowing ability. Am J Phys Med Rehabil, n.95, p.270-276, 2016.

TAKAHASHI, K.; GROHER, M. E.; MICHI, K. Methodology for detecting swallowing sounds. Dysphagia, n.9, p.54-62, 1994.

TAYLOR KJW, BURNS P, WELLS PNT. Clinical applications of Doppler ultrasound. In: FRIEDMAN LS Gastrointestinal Unit. Raven Press. New York, p.415, 1995.

VASCONCELOS, R. L. M.; MOURA, T. L.; CAMPOS, T. F.; LINDQUIST, A. R. R.; GUERRA, R. O. Evaluation of the functional performance of children with cerebral palsy according to levels of motor impairment. Rev Bras Fisioter, n.13, v.5, p.390-397, 2009.

VIANA, C. I. O.; SUZUKI, H. S. Cerebral palsy: analysis of swallowing patterns before and after speech therapy intervention. Rev CEFAC, n.13, v.5, p.790-800, 2011.

VIVONE, G. P.; TAVARES, M. M. M.; BARTOLOMEU, R. S.; NEMR, K.; CHIAPPETTA, A. L. M. L. Analysis of eating consistency and swallowing time in children with spastic quadriplegic cerebral palsy. Rev. CEFAC, n.4, v.9, p.504-511, 2007.

WEIR, K. A. M. C.; MAHON, S.; TAYLOR, S.; CHANG, A. B. Oropharyngeal aspiration and silent aspiration in children. CHEST, n. 140 v.3, p. 589-597, 2011.

WRIGHT, R. E. R.; WRIGHT, F. R.; CARSON, C. A. Videofluoroscopic assessment in children with severe cerebral palsy presenting with dysphagia. Paediatr Radiot, n.26, p.720-722, 1996.

YOUMANS, S. R.; STIERWALT, J. A. G. An acoustic profile of normal swallowing. Dysphagia, n. 20, p. 195-209, 2005.

ZAGZEBSKI, J. A. Physics and instrumentation in Doppler and B-mode ultrasound. In: ZWIELBEL, WL. Introduction to vascular ultrasound, Revinter.3 ed. Rio de Janeiro, 1996.

DOCUMENTS CONSULTED

ARAUJO, B. C. L. Accuracy of clinical diagnosis of dysphagia in children with cerebral palsy. Dissertation (Master's in Child and Adolescent Health) - Federal University of Pernambuco, Recife, p. 78, 2012.

ASSIS-MADEIRA, E. A.; CARVALHO, S. G.; BLASCOVI-ASSIS, S. M. Functional performance of children with cerebral palsy from high and low socioeconomic levels. Rev Paul Pediatr, n.31, v.1, p. 51-57, 2013.

CANS, C. Surveillance of cerebral palsy in Europe: a collaboration of cerebral palsy surveys and registers. Dev Med Child Neurol, n.42, p.816-824, 2000.

CHAGAS, P. S. C.; DEFILIPO, E. C.; LEMOS, R. A.; MANCINI, M. C.; FRÔNIO, J. S.; CARVALHO, R. M. Classification of motor function and functional performance of children with cerebral palsy. Rev Bras Fisioter, n.12, v.5, p.409-416, 2008.

CLAVÉ, P.; TERRÉ, R.; KRAA, M.; SERRA, M. Attitude to follow in the face of oropharyngeal dysphagia. Rev Esp Enferm Dig, n.2, v.96, 2004.

ERASMUS, C. E.; HULST, K. V.; ROTTEVEEL, J. J.; ILLEMSEN, M. A. A. P.; JONGERIUS, P. H. Swallowing problems in cerebral palsy. Eur J Paediatr, n. 171, p.409-414, 2012.

JAHNSEN, R.; AAMODT, G.; ROSENBAUM, P. Gross motor function classification system used in adults with cerebral palsy: agreement of self reported versus professional rating. Dev Med Child Neurol, n.48, p.734-738, 2006.

JALIL, A. A. A.; KATZKA, D. A.; CASTELL, D. O. Approach to the patient with dysphagia. The American Journal of Medicine, n.128, v.10, p.1138.e17- 1138.e23, 2015.

JIMENEZ, D. G.; MARTIN, J. J. D.; GARCIA, C. B.; TREVINO, S. J. Gastrointestinal pathology in children with infantile cerebral palsy and other neurological disabilities. An Pediatr, n.73, v.6, p.361-366, 2010.

LEE, K. D.; SONG, S. H.; KOO, J. H.; PARK, H. S.; KIM, J. S.; JANG, K. H. Proposed Use of Thickener According to Fluid Intake on Videofluoroscopic Swallowing Studies: Preliminary Study in Normal Healthy Persons. Ann Rehabil Med, n. 40, v. 2, p. 206-213, 2016.

MANCINI, M. C.; ALVES, A. C. M.; SCHAPER, C.; FIGUEIREDO, E. M.; SAMPAIO, R. F.; COELHO, Z. A. C.; TIRADO, M. G. A. Cerebral palsy severity and functional performance. Rev. Bras. Fisioter, n. 8, v. 3, p. 253-260, 2004.

MILLER, C. L. Aspiration and swallowing dysfunction in paediatrics patients. ICAN: Infant, child and adolescent nutrition, n.3, v.6, p. 336-343, 2011.

MOLFENTER, SM; STEELE, CM. Temporal variability in the deglutition literature. Dysphagia, n.27, v.2, p.162-177, 2012.

PANETH, N.; QIU, H.; ROSENBAUM, P.; SAIGAL, S.; BISHAI, S.; JETTON, J.; OUDEN, L. D.; BROYLES, S.; TYSON, J.; KUGLER, K. Reliability of classification of cerebral palsy in low-birthweight in children in four countries. Dev Med Child Neurol, n. 45, p. 628-633, 2003.

SILVA, M. C. F.; FRIEDMAN, S. Analysis of Brazilian speech therapy scientific production on cerebral palsy. Rev Soc Bras Fonoaudiol, n. 15, v. 4, p.589-593, 2010.

ANNEXES

ANNEX 1 - INFORMED CONSENT FORM
Project Title: COMPARATIVE ANALYSIS OF DEGLUTATION SOUNDS IN CHILDREN WITH CEREBRAL PARALYSIS AND NORMAL CHILDREN EVALUATED WITH DOPPLER DURANE SONAR CLINICAL AND VIDEOFLUOROSCOPIC EVALUATION
Researcher: Fga. Liliane de F. Friedrich Gallinea

Place of Research: CRAID (Regional Centre for the Care of the Disabled) and HOSPITAL DE CLINICAS / UFPR

Address and telephone (mobile): Estrada da Sereia, 5750 - (41) 9 8836-4602

PURPOSE OF PATIENT INFORMATION AND CONSENT DOCUMENT

Your child is being invited to take part in a survey. The information in this document is intended to help you fully understand the aims of the research, and to let you know that your participation is spontaneous. If you have any questions while reading this document, you should ask so that you can fully understand what it is all about. Once you have been informed about the following information, if you agree to take part in the study, please sign this document, which is in two copies, one for you and one for the researcher in charge.

INTRODUCTION:

For a child to grow and develop properly, it's not enough for them to be given the right foods. They must be able to chew and swallow them properly. Many children with neurological problems don't have this ability, so they quickly become malnourished and dehydrated and even aspirate their own saliva, causing repeated pneumonia, because the child may be suffering from dysphagia. Dysphagia is a disorder that requires the patient to receive a correct diagnosis, treatment and monitoring for proper progression. Difficulties in swallowing in children with neurological disorders have been shown to be important, and research reinforces the need for instrumental swallowing assessments, so that the most appropriate clinical and speech therapy treatment can be carried out for each child.

PURPOSE OF THE RESEARCH:

To analyse the sounds of swallowing in children with cerebral palsy and in children without neuromotor alterations, using Doppler sonar (equipment that can pick up sounds in the body, used in pregnant women to listen to the baby's heart) and videofluoroscopy.

PROCEDURE:

To do this, samples need to be taken. This is done through a clinical assessment in which the speech therapist will ask you a few questions about your diet.

Afterwards, your child will undergo a swallowing test called videofluoroscopy, which will be carried out on the X-ray machine, where you will eat a water content thickened with cornstarch, plus a barium gel contrast product, allowing the child to swallow.

we can visualise how your child eats. During the examination, a small piece of equipment will be placed on the side of your neck, without any pressure, to capture the sound of swallowing.

DISCOMFORT:

There is no discomfort during the examination, but you will be exposed to a small dose of radiation during the swallowing assessment procedure (Videofluoroscopy), with a maximum exposure time of 2 minutes. The examination will be carried out by a doctor and speech therapist researchers Rosane Sampaio Santos, Edna Márcia and Liliane de F. Friedrich Galeria at the Hospital de Clínicas and CRAID (Regional Centre for Assistance to the Disabled). The test does not require anaesthetic. The person being tested may experience constipation after the test, due to ingestion of cornstarch with water and barium.

COSTS:

You won't have to pay for the survey.

PARTICIPATION:

If your child wishes to withdraw from taking part in the research, they can do so at any time. Your participation is voluntary.

All research participants will be informed, monitored and treated by the researcher: Liliane de Fátima Friedrich Gallinea, speech therapist, graduated from the Catholic University of Paraná, CRFa-5819, resident: Estrada da Sereia, 5750, Campo Largo - phone: (41) 8836-4602. During the course of the research, should you or your child have any questions or need any further guidance, please use the telephone number above.

PRIVACY AND CONFIDENTIALITY:

You have been given an undertaking by the researchers that your image and identity will be kept strictly confidential. All data will be kept confidential. In all records, a code will replace your child's name. The data collected will be used to evaluate the study, and may also be used in scientific publications about this study. However, your child's identity will not be revealed under any circumstances.

RESPONSIBILITY:

In the event of new information during the course of the research, it will be submitted to the Ethics Committee for a new opinion.

DECLARATION OF CONSENT:

I, ____ , bearer of ID: ________________________________ I, the undersigned, agree to allow my son (daughter) to   participate in the study described above.

I have been duly informed and clarified by the researcher, Liliane de F. Friedrich Gallinea and Rosane Sampaio Santos, who are responsible for this study, about the procedures involved, as well as the possible risks and benefits arising from my child's participation. I have been assured that I am free to accept or refuse to allow my child to take part in this research, and that I can withdraw my consent at any time, without this leading to any penalty or interruption of my monitoring/assistance/treatment. I agree that the data collected for the study will be used for the purpose described above.

I have understood the information presented in this consent form and have had the opportunity to be properly informed.

I will receive a signed and dated copy of this Informed Consent Document.

Curitiba,___/___/___.

____

Patient's name

Signature of Patient or Guardian

Researcher's name

Researcher's signature

ANNEX 2 - SWALLOWING CLINICAL ASSESSMENT PROTOCOL

SWALLOWING CLINICAL ASSESSMENT PROTOCOL

1. IDENTIFICATION:

Patient	
Age	
Date of Birth	
Sex	□ Male □ Female
Diagnosis	
Type and location of injury	
Time of injury	
Associated pathologies	
Have you ever had speech therapy	□ Yes □ NoStimulation time:
Referral	

2. CLINICAL ASPECTS:

Clinical history	

Apgar	1º minute: 5º minute: 10th minute:
Date of Birth	
Sex	□ Male □ Female
Medication	
BCP	□ Yes□ NoHow many :
Nutritional status (weight curve)	□ Nourished □ Malnourished
Feeding route	□ Oral□ SNG□ SNE□ SOG □Gastrostomy DJejunostomy □ Parenteral
Breathing	□ DOxygen-dependent environment□ VM □ Use of NIMV Tracheostomy: □ Cuff: □ Inflated UPacially Inflated □ Deflated Speech valve: □ Yes□ No

3. CONSCIENCE:

Responsive	□ **Under 15** '□ **Over 15'**

4. COGNITIVE:

Skill s age-appropriate communication	□ Yes□ No

5. OBSERVATION AT REST

Age-appropriate cervical control:	□ Yes□ NoHow many :
Presence of pathological reflexes:	□ Yes□ NoWhat :
Posture:	□ Supine position □ Sitting 45°□ Sitting 90° Need adaptations: □ No □ Yes Which ones:
Breathing:	□ Noisy □ Oral □ NasalDTachypnoea Dyspnoea
Lip sealing:	□ Efficient □ Not efficient
Tongue posture:	□ NDN□ Protrusion
Sialorrhoea:	□ Yes□ No
Nasal reflux:	□ Yes□ No
Jaw:	□ Efficient □ Not efficient
Saliva stasis in the oral cavity:	□ Present □ Absent
Cervical auscultation:	□ Positive □ Negative

6. SPONTANEOUS SWALLOWING:

Clinical signs of aspiration:	Cough□Dyspnoea □ Wet voice
If tracheostomised:	Blue Dye Test: □ Positive□ Negative
Cervical auscultation:	□ Positive□ Negative

7. STRUCTURAL ASSESSMENT:

Facial symmetry		□ Yes□ NoHow many :
Teething	Erupted teeth	
	Type of bite	□ Open □Overjet□Overbite□ Normal
	Occlusion	□ Class I □ Class II □ Class III □Angle
	Oral Hygiene	□ BEG□ REG□ PEG
Sensitivity	Facial	□ Normal□ Altered □ Decreased□ Exacerbated
	Language	□ Normal□ Altered □ Decreased□ Exacerbated
Oral reflexes	Searching	□ Present□ Absent□ Exacerbated

	Suction	□ Present□	Absent□	Exacerbated
	From Bite	□ Present□	Absent□	Exacerbated
	Vomit	□ Present□	Absent□	Exacerbated
Isolated Mobility	Language	□ Efficient □ Not efficient		
	Lips	□ Efficient □ Not efficient		
	Cheek	□ Efficient □ Not efficient		
	Jaw	□ Efficient □ Not efficient		
	Tongue strength	□ Efficient □ Not efficient		

8. VOCAL ASSESSMENT

Voluntary coughing	□ Yes□ No
Vocal quality	□ SoprosityURoquidãoU Aspereza □ Wet voice
Vocal intensity	□ Normal □ Reduced □ Increased
Resonance	□ HypernasalUHyponasalU Normal
After swallowing saliva	□ Normal □ Wet voice

9. FUNCTIONAL FOOD EVALUATION

Conditions in the evaluation of *the* diet offer		
Position	□ sitting 90° □ sitting 45°	
	With adaptations: □ Yes □ NoWhat:	
Diet offered	Liquid: □ WaterQuantity in ml: □ Juice Quantity in ml: □ MilkQuantity in ml:	
	Nectar	□ 200 ml liquid+10 g commercial thickener (2 sachets)
	Mel	□ for 200 ml liquid+12.5 g thickener (2 $/^1_2$ sachets)
	Pudding	□ 200 ml liquid+15 g thickener (3 sachets)
	Solid	□ biscuit (like a social club)
Utensils	□ Cup □ Spoon □ Syringe □ Bottle	
Observation of the patient's diet	Anticipatory phase	Feeds itself: □ Yes □ No Efficient :□ Yes □ No With adaptations :□ No □ Yes Which ones:

9.5 Consistencies and findings of the clinical assessment of swallowing

	Consistency	Liquid	Nectar	Mel	Pudding
Volume					
Number of swallows					
Capturing the cake					
Lip sealing					
Preparing the cake					
Extra-oral exhaust					
Transit time					
Oral and pharyngeal coordination					
Residues in the oral cavity after swallowing					
Laryngeal elevation					
Clinical signs of aspiration					
Aspiration					
Cough reflex					
Dyspnoea					
Wet voice					
Pigarette					
Discomfort					

10-PROGNOSIS:

<table>
<tr><td></td></tr>
<tr><td></td></tr>
</table>

11.COMMENTS/DESCRIPTION:

<table>
<tr><td></td></tr>
<tr><td></td></tr>
<tr><td></td></tr>
</table>

12.HANDLING:

<table>
<tr><td></td></tr>
<tr><td></td></tr>
<tr><td></td></tr>
</table>

ANNEX 3- PROTOCOL FOR ASSESSING SWALLOWING USING VIDEOFLUOROSCOPY

SWALLOWING VIDEOFLUOROSCOPY PROTOCOL

1. **IDENTIFICATION:**

Patient	
Age	
Date of Birth	
Sex	□ Male □ Female
Diagnosis	
Type and location of injury	
Time of injury	
Associated pathologies	
Have you ever had speech therapy	□ Yes□ NoStimulation time:
Referral	

2. **GENERAL STATUS**

Level of consciousness	□ AlertaUTorporoso
Understanding verbal commands	□ Yes □ No □ Partial
Collaborative	□ Yes □ No
Glasgow	□1□2□3□4□5□6□7□8□9□10 □ 11 □ 12 □ 13 □ 14 □ 15 □ NA
Medications	

3. **DENTITION**

Teething	□ Complete	□ In complete

4. RESPIRATORY CONDITIONS

Oxygen-dependent	□ Yes □ No
Tracheostomy	□ Yes □ No Cuff: □ Inflated □ Partially inflated □ Deflated
Mechanical ventilation	□ Yes □ No
Non-invasive mechanical ventilation	□ Yes □ No
Speech valve	□ Yes □ No Time:

5. FOOD

Feeding route	□ Oral□ SNG□ SNE□ SOG □Gastrostomy □Jejunostomy □ Parenteral

6. CONSISTENCIES OFFERED IN THE EXAM

Diet offered	Liquid	□ 70 ml of water and 30 ml of GuedertCp barium
	Pasty	□ 70 ml of water and 30ml of Guedert barium and 5g of thickenerCp
	Pasty	□ 70 ml of water and 30ml of Guedert barium and 10g of
	thick	thickenerCp
	Solid	□3 biscuits (social club type) soaked in GuedertCp barium

7. CONDITIONS FOR EXAMINING AND OFFERING THE DIET

Position	□ sitting 90° □ sitting 45°
	With adaptations: □ Yes □ NoWhat:
Utensils	□ Cup □ Spoon □ Syringe □ Bottle □ Straw
Incidence	□ Profile□ Posterior anterus □ right oblique□ left oblique

8. CONSISTENCIES AND EXAMINATION FINDINGS

	Free Sip	Solid	Pasty	Thin Pasty	Liquid
Oral Phase	Capturing the Cake				
	Lip sealing				
	Cake positioning				
	Extra oral exhaust				
	Preparation/mastication				
	Oral Ejection				
	Oral/Pharyngeal Phase Coordination				
	Residues in the Oral Cavity				
Pharyngeal phase	Velopharyngeal seal				
	Laryngeal penetration				
	Tracheal suction				
	Residues in pharyngeal recesses				
	Vallecules				
	Pharyngeal wall				
	Piriform recesses				
	Asymmetry in the descent through the pharynx				

CAPTION: E = EFFICIENT; NE = NOT EFFICIENT, P= PRESENT, A = ABSENT, T = LATE; 1, 2, 3 = NUMBER OF SWALLOWS

9. CONSISTENCIES AND EXAMINATION FINDINGS

	SOLID	PASTY	FINE PASTRY	LIQUID

		3ml	5ml	10ml	3ml	5ml	10ml	3ml	5ml	10ml
Oral Phase	Capturing the Cake									
	Lip sealing									
	Cake positioning									
	Extra oral exhaust									
	Preparation/mastication									
	Oral Ejection									
	Oral/Pharyngeal Phase Coordination									
	Oral residue after swallowing									
Pharyngeal phase	Velopharyngeal sealing									
	Laryngeal penetration									
	Tracheal suction									
	Residues in pharyngeal recesses									
	Vallecules									
	Pharyngeal wall									
	Piriform recesses									
	Asymmetry in the descent through the pharynx									

10. ESOPHAGIC PHASE

CLASSIFICATION OF DYSPHAGIA SEVERITY BY VIDEOFLUOROSCOPY

☐ **Normal swallowing**

Mild dysphagia: altered oral control, delayed pharyngeal response, little residue, no laryngotracheal penetration or aspiration.

☐ **Moderate dysphagia**: poor oral control, pharyngeal residue in all consistencies and poor laryngotracheal aspiration of one consistency.

Severe dysphagia: presence of substantial laryngotracheal aspiration or when the patient fails to swallow.

CONCLUSION:

ANNEX 4 - ORAL INTAKE SCALE

FUNCTIONAL ORAL INTAKE SCALE (FOIS) CRARY & GROHER (2005)

Patient	
Sex	□ Male □ Female

Level 1	□ Nothing by mouth
Level 2	□ Dependent on alternative and minimal oral route of some food or liquid
Level 3	□ Dependent on alternative route with consistent oral route of food or liquid
Level 4	□ Total oral route of a single consistency.
Level 5	Total oral route with multiple consistencies, but with the need for special preparation or compensations.
Level 6	Total oral route with multiple consistencies, but without the need for special preparation or compensations, but with dietary restrictions.
Level 7	□ Full motorway without restrictions.

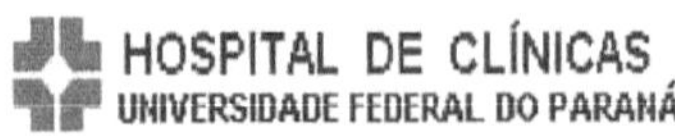

2ª VIA

Curitiba, 12 de março de 2010.

Ilmo (a) Sr. (a)
Liliane de Fátima Friedrich Gallinea
Neste

Prezada Pesquisadora:

    Comunicamos que o Projeto de Pesquisa intitulado "ANALISE COMPARATIVA DOS SONS DA DEGLUTIÇÃO EM CRIANÇAS COM PARALISIA CEREBRAL E CRIANÇAS NORMAIS AVALIADAS COM SONAR DOPPLER", foi analisado com pendências, pelo Comitê de Ética em Pesquisa em Seres Humanos, em reunião realizada no dia 24 de novembro de 2009. Após atendimento das pendências pelo Pesquisador, consideramos o projeto aprovado em 12 de março de 2010. O referido projeto atende aos aspectos das Resoluções CNS 196/96, e demais, sobre Diretrizes e Normas Regulamentadoras de Pesquisa Envolvendo Seres Humanos do Ministério da Saúde.

CAAE: 0278.0.208.000-09
Registro CEP: 2099.266/2009-11

Conforme a Resolução 196/96, solicitamos que sejam apresentados a este CEP, relatórios sobre o andamento da pesquisa, bem como informações relativas às modificações do protocolo, cancelamento, encerramento e destino dos conhecimentos obtidos.

Data para entrega do primeiro relatório: 12 de setembro de 2010.

Atenciosamente,

Renato Tambara Filho
Coordenador do Comitê de Ética em Pesquisa
em Seres Humanos do Hospital de Clinicas/UFPR

ACADEMIC PRODUCTION

Article submitted to the Brazilian Journal of Otorhinolaryngology BJORL.

A COMPARATIVE ANALYSIS OF SWALLOWING SOUNDS IN CHILDREN WITH AND WITHOUT CEREBRAL PALSY USING SONAR DOPPLER: A PRELIMINARY STUDY

A COMPARATIVE ANALYSIS OF SWALLOWING SOUNDS IN CHILDREN WITH AND WITHOUT CEREBRAL PALSY USING DOPPLER SONAR: A PRELIMINARY STUDY

Liliane de Fátima Friedrich Gallinea[1] , Edna Marcia Abdulmasshin[2] , Rosane Sampaio Santos[3] , GiselaCarmona Hirata[4] , Cibele Fontoura Cagliari[5] , Mônica Nunes Lima Cat[6] , Adriane Celli

[1]Child and Adolescent Master's degree student, Department of Paediatrics and

Otorhinolaryngology Department, Dysphagia Division, Hospital de Clínicas, UFPR, Curitiba/ PR, Brazil. [2] Phd, Otorhinolaryngology Department, Dysphagia Division, Hospital de Clínicas, UFPR, Curitiba/PR, Brazil.

[3] Phd, Otorhinolaryngology Department, Dysphagia Division, Hospital de Clínicas, UFPR, Curitiba/PR, Brazil.

[4]Dysphagia Division, Master of Communication Disorders, University Tuiuti of Paraná, Curitiba/PR, Brazil.

[5]Dysphagia Division, Master of Communication Disorders, University Tuiuti of Paraná, Curitiba/PR, Brazil.

[6]Phd, Department of Pediatrics, Children and Adolescent Health Post Graduation Division, Hospital de Clínicas, UFPR, Curitiba/PR, Brazil.

[7]Phd, Department of Pediatrics, Child and Adolescent Health Post Graduation Division, and Pediatric Gastroenterology Division, Hospital de Clínicas, UFPR, Curitiba/ PR, Brazil.

Address for correspondence with the author: Liliane de Fátima Friedrich Gallinea

5750, Estrada da Sereia- zip code: 83607.310 - Curitiba - PR- Brazil

Email: lilianef. gallinea@gmail.com

There is no conflict of interest.

Keywords: cerebral palsy, deglutition disorders, dysphagia, swallowing sounds, sonar Doppler.

Abstract

Introduction: Dysphagia, frequently accompanied by aspiration, is a common symptom in children with cerebral palsy. Using sonar Doppler to capture swallowing sounds of children with and without oropharyngeal dysphagia and comparing the sound patterns obtained from the two groups, one may evaluate whether the use of sonar Doppler could potentially be an effective non-invasive alternative for diagnosing pharyngeal dysphagia by determining whether the disorder causes measurable differences in the sound patterns produced during swallowing.

Objective: The aim of this study was to use sonar Doppler and videofluoroscopy to determine whether any significant difference exists between the swallowing sounds of children with and without cerebral palsy.

Methods: A case-control study was conducted in order to evaluate the swallowing sounds of 21 children with cerebral palsy and 21 children without neuromotor impairment. The sounds were captured using Doppler sonar during a simultaneous videofluoroscopy study.

Results: Swallowing duration was significantly longer in the cerebral palsy group for both food consistencies. Significant differences between the two groups were seen for all three variables evaluated when fed the liquid food consistency. The groups exhibited significant differences for two of the variables when fed the nectar food consistency.

Conclusion: The data seem to suggest that the swallowing process in cerebral palsy patients, in addition to being slower than that of patients without neuromotor impairment, produces differences in the sound patterns which could indicate the presence of oropharyngeal dysphagia, as a result of abnormalities in muscle tone and movement found in children with the disorder. However, although the study was able to determine significant differences in sonar Doppler assessment of children with cerebral palsy, it was unable to detect a wave pattern suggesting aspiration or penetration. A large group study or alternative methods of sound-signal analysis are needed in order to address this issue.

Introduction

The act of swallowing naturally involves a large number of oral and pharyngeal muscles working together in a perfectly synchronised manner, stopping the breathing process and protecting the respiratory tract. Dysphagia denotes a dysfunction of the oral cavity, the pharynx, the esophagus, or the esophagogastric junction which may cause food to enter the respiratory tract, resulting in coughing, suffocation/asphyxia, lung disorders, and aspiration.[1,2]It is a common symptom in children with cerebral palsy, and problems such as regurgitation, malnutrition, growth deficiency, constant coughing during and/or after feeding, and chronic lung disease with recurrent prandial aspiration are often reported by parents and caregivers.

Children with cerebral palsy frequently display symptoms such as the following: inability to control food in the mouth, loss of mobility in both the upper and lower lips, lack of lip competence due to insufficient strength, lack of or exaggeration of oral reflexes, premature anterior escape of food, lack of tongue control for either front-to-back or side-to -side motion, alterations of the orofacial muscles with a loss of intraoral pressure,inadequate propulsion of the bolus, presence of intraoral food residue, and pharyngeal alterations such as a delay in the triggering of the swallowing reflex, premature spillage of bolus into pharynx, diminished pharyngeal peristalsis, alterations in the elevation and contraction of the larynx, presence of residue in the epiglotticvalleculae and piriform sinuses, motility disorder of the cricopharyngeus muscle, or the occurrence of respiration before, during, or after swallowing.The disorder is also associated with nutritional deficiencies, weight loss,dehydration, regurgitation, occurrence of coughing while eating, occurrence of a "gurgly" voice, dyspnea,or an increase in secretions from the upper respiratory tract. As a result, patients with dysphagia have a high risk of developing recurrent pneumonia and malnutrition.[3-12]

The methods currently used to evaluate, diagnose, and monitor dysphagia in children with cerebral palsy include cervical auscultation,[13-15] fibre-optic endoscopic evaluation of swallowing (FEES)[16] and a videofluoroscopy swallowing study (VFSS).[4,6,8,17-21] The videofluoroscopy swallowing study (VFSS) is considered the gold standard, but it has several drawbacks, such as exposing children to radiation, requiring highly trained professionals and rooms with specialised equipment. Furthermore, in Brazil these studies are usually only performed in a few tertiary hospitals or specialised clinics, resulting in a long waiting list for children who rely on public health services, as they are not widely available.Although cervical auscultation using a stethoscope is non-invasive, its limitations include a lack of standardised measurements and a reliance on subjective sound descriptions. The neck region produces a significant amount of acoustic activity, and understanding the sounds produced during swallowing is a complex task. Sounds generated as a result of pathological swallowing need to be identified and studied more closely in order to identify acoustic parameters that may be quantified and measured, thereby allowing one to objectively evaluate the swallowing sounds that may indicate whether or not pharyngeal dysphagia and/or aspiration is in fact present.Other non-invasive procedures (including the use of an accelerometer and microphone) used to evaluate both normal and pathological deglutition based on swallowing sounds have already been described.[22,23]

HAMLET describes the most prominent acoustic feature of the swallowing sound as being the movement of the bolus through the pharynx and the upper oesophageal sphincter. A periodic noise, perhaps from the larynx, "explodes," creating an acoustic signal in which the closure of the cricopharyngeus muscle figures most prominently. Hyoid, laryngeal and epiglotticmotion also contribute to the acoustic swallowing pattern. Thus, normal swallowing consists of an audible double click.[22,23]CICHERO & MURDOCH described the three components which they perceived to be responsible for the swallowing sound - the first corresponds to a weak signal associated with elevation and forward excursion of the larynx,as well as the passage of the bolus through the pharynx;the second is a strong sound associated with the opening of the upper cricopharyngeus sphincter, and the third, a weak signal associated with the descent of the larynx after swallowing.[24]Based on these studies, a normality pattern of the swallowing sounds of 50 healthy adults was generated using Doppler sonar and described by Santos.[25] The same parameters have also been studied in healthy children by Cagliari.[26]
The development of a new technique for detecting and analysing swallowing sounds using sonar Doppler would offer speech therapists a useful and accessible tool for objectively monitoring their patients, which could serve as an alternative to the subjective cervical auscultation technique. It must be emphasised that the use of the sonar Doppler enables one to evaluate swallowing without exposing the patient to radiation or subjecting him to other invasive methods. Furthermore, the sonar Doppler device is portable and easily transported to institutions,schools, or a private bedside. For these reasons, sonar Doppler could potentially be an effective, non-invasive method for assessing aspiration in cerebral palsy patients.
The aim of the present study was to compare swallowing sounds using sonar Doppler in children with and without cerebral palsy in order to determine whether any difference exists between the parameters of the swallowing sounds of children who do not suffer from other neurological pathology or dysphagia and those of children with cerebral palsy who also exhibit dysphagia. The sonar Doppler findings were correlated with thoseof the videofluoroscopy study in order to determine whether it is possible to identify any acoustic characteristic which may indicate the occurrence of bronchoaspiration using sonar Doppler.

Materials and Methods

Design: A case-control study was conducted in order to evaluate the swallowing sounds of 21 children with cerebral palsy and 21 children without neuromotor impairment, paired according to gender and age (ranging from 2-15 years of age). The sounds were captured using Doppler sonar during a simultaneous videofluoroscopy study (VFSS).

Participants:The study group consisted of 21 children, aged between 2 and 15 years, 8 of which (38%) were females and 13(62%) males. All patients had been diagnosed with cerebral palsy and referred for videofluoroscopy studies (VFSS) due to complaints of dysphagia. The patients were submitted to both clinical and instrumental swallowing evaluations consisting of a videofluoroscopy and simultaneous sonar Doppler analysis.The control group, whose acoustic data was also taken using sonar Doppler, consisted of 21 childrenwithout neuromotor impairment and without symptoms of dysphagia, paired according to age and gender with the children with cerebral palsy. The control group was not studied directly by all the authors of the present article, but rather consists of data from children who were part of a previous study carried out by the researcher CibeleFontoura Cagliari.[26] Exclusion criteria for the group of children with cerebral palsyincluded the following: previous prohibition of oral intake and lack of cooperation, (for example, constant crying during the sonar Doppler evaluations).This study had the approval of the Ethics Committee, registration number CEP: 2099.2566/2009-11, March, 12th 2010. All parents or guardians responsible for the children who participated in the study signed the informed consent forms under registration number CEP: 2099.266/2009-11.

Assessment: All participants were assessed using a clinical evaluation, videofluoroscopy (VFSS) and sonar Doppler. Clinical evaluation included analysis of medical history and both a structural and functional evaluation of the swallowing.Using sonar Doppler, swallowing sounds were recorded simultaneously with the feeding of the sample or modified food for the VFSS. The sound patterns were recorded and analysed using Voxmetria software.[27]

VFSS Equipment: Siemens Axiom model R100® X-ray machine and Siemens monitor model M44-2® were used to perform the videofluoroscopy swallowing study. Images were digitised on the HP Pavilion TX 2075BR laptop using the TV capture card USB Sapphire Wonder TV.

VFSS Procedures: During the assessment, patients were seated in a chair adapted for the purpose and adjusted to 90 degrees with a lateral radiographic view. [4,6,8,17-21,28]The food consistencies used for the joint VFSS and sonar Doppler sound capture studies were nectar (thin puree), pudding (thick puree), and liquid, according to the American Dietetic Association nomenclature.[29] To obtain these consistencies the researchers used 70% water mixed with Barium Sulfate 100% from Bariogel (as a radiological contrast, containing 1 g barium sulfate and 1 ml gsp vehicle for paediatric and adult use) and a modified instant cornstarch food thickenerof the brand Thick&Easy (composed of modified cornstarch - E1442, maltodextrin, tara gum, xanthan gum and guar gum). According to the nutritional information given by the product, each 100gcontained375 kcal, 100gof carbohydrates,and 125 mg of sodium. Using the preparation methods and consistency indications as given in the manufacturar's instructions,5ml of each consistency was prepared andfed to the child, and at least three swallows of each texturewere recorded during a 2 minuteinterval [15]. Feeding utensils available were a cup, spoon, plastic syringe, and the child's bottle, used only when necessary.The choice of these consistencies was not random, but rather was due to the great difficulty in eating that most of the children in the study group experienced. These three consistencies - nectar (thin puree), pudding (thick puree), and liquid - were the most readily accepted by this group and therefore the best suited for capturing swallowing sounds.

In addition to the researchers/speech-language pathologists and one professor/speech-language pathologist with who is both experienced and certified in conducting the VFSS, those present comprised a radiologist (to operate the equipment and controlling the dosage and radiation exposure time), and the mother, father, or caregiver who accompanied the child during the exam and normally assisted with the feeding.The caregiver related the child's feeding preferences, the consistencies normally offered daily, and any precautions used during feeding. Adequate safety equipment was used during the VFSS exams, including a vest and lead thyroid protector, safety goggles, and disposable gloves, used by the professionals and parents present during the exam for offering the food sample containing the barium.

VFSS Analysis: Evaluation of the oral phase considered lip closure, anterior premature spillage, multiple swallows, insufficient bolus formation, prolonged oral time, presence of oral cavity residue, and reduced tongue movements.Disorders involving the pharyngeal phase include a delayed or absent swallow reflex, delayed triggering of the pharyngeal swallow, premature spillage of the bolus into the pharynx, uncoordinated pharyngeal contraction, penetration or aspiration before, during, or after swallowing, and reduced laryngeal elevation.Evaluation during the pharyngeal phase considered delayed triggering of the pharyngeal swallow, contrast passing through pharynx, pharyngeal residue (in the valleculae and piriform sinuses), hyoid motion, laryngeal penetration, and tracheal aspiration. Also evaluated were cricopharyngeus muscle opening, cricopharyngeus bar, and protection of the upper airway such as larynx elevation and closure.Laryngeal penetration and tracheal aspiration were thoroughly evaluated before, during and after swallowing. Evaluation of the oesophageal phase considered information such as oesophageal peristalsis clearance, opening of the inferior oesophageal sphincter, and the presence of gastroesophageal reflux.[4,6,8,17-21,28]

Thevideofluoroscopy features were evaluatedaccording to the classification of dysphagia severity described by Ott et al, whichclassifies dysphagia as either mild, moderate, or severe. If the child demonstrated difficulty in oral control, a delayed pharyngeal response, presence of little residue, but no penetration or tracheal aspiration, the dysphagia was classified as mild. If the child demonstrated poor oral control, presence of pharyngeal residue for all consistencies, but little penetration or tracheal aspiration of one consistency, his dysphagia was classified as moderate; however, if substantial tracheal aspirationwas observed, the child's dysphagia was classified as severe.[30] VFSS images were recorded, analysed and compared to the swallowing sounds captured by the Doppler sonar.The parents and/or caregivers who participated in the VFSS and sonar Doppler studies received a report with the results of instrumental evaluation of the swallowing according to the videofluoroscopy study (VFSS), informing them of the level of severity of the dysphagia according to OTT classification: normal swallowing, mild dysphagia, moderate dysphagia, and severe dysphagia, based on the oral and pharyngeal difficulties observed and the presence or absence of laryngotracheal aspiration.[30]The report explained for which food consistencies the difficulties were observed.Given the difficulty in feeding the children of the study group (as most children were tetraplegic with oropharyngeal dysphagia,lacked functional mastication patterns, and were unaccustomed to solid food intake), solid food was not used in VFSS testing. The researchers opted for evaluation of swallowing sounds produced using liquid and nectar consistencies only since they were more readily accepted by the entire study group.

VFSS image with concomitant use of Sonar Doppler to capture the sounds of swallowing.Demonstrating oral phase, liquid suction in the bottle, in a child with cerebral palsy, with oropharyngeal dysphagia.

Sonar Doppler Equipment: The continuous-wave Doppler equipment used to capture the swallowing sounds was a portable ultrasonic detector (model DF - 4001 Martec) with a flat disc transducer and single crystal, providing the interface to the Doppler. The frequency of the Doppler ultrasounds was 2.5 MHz, with an output of $10mW/cm^2$, and power sound output was 1W. The equipment was attached to a standard HP Pavilion 2075 BR TX laptop computer whose operating system was Windows Vista Home Premium. During the VFSS and sonar Doppler examinations, each patient was seated with the head in neutral alignment. The sonar Doppler transducer was placed on the right side of the neck on the lateral portion of the trachea, just below the cricoid cartilage, as described by Takahashi, Groher and Michi as the best place for cervical auscultation.[31] The beam of ultrasonic energy emitted by the transducer was positioned to form an angle of 30°- 60°. Contact® gel was used in order to decrease ultrasound dispersion into the air and increase its body transmission and echo, favouring the acoustic signal recording.[31,32]

Figure 1- Sonar Doppler equipment used during the research to capture the sounds of swallowing.

Acoustic analysis of the swallowing sounds: The sound patterns were recorded and later analysed using the 2.8 version of VoxMetria software (developed by CTS Computers), and further elaborated using the method previously described by BEHLAU & MICHAELIS[27] , allowing an accurate measurement. This software has the capacity to process sounds produced by swallowing and represent them visually in wave format, depicting intensity, frequency and time.[22-26, 33-35] After recording each individual's name, age, and address, the researcher created a sound file for later analysis. The software's voice analysis function was chosen to record the swallowing sound using the following parameters: audio signal, intensity, and fundamental frequency. The volume of the sonar Doppler device was adjusted to number 1 for more effective capture of the audio signal by the VoxMetria programme and lower external noise interference.

Acoustic Parameters:The data from the sound patterns of the swallowing were analysed and classified as previously described by Santos and Macedo[25] , Abdulmassih et al[35] : a) Initial Frequency (IF) of the sound wave - frequency at the beginning of the acoustic signal measured in Hz. b) Peak Frequency (PF) of the sound wave - frequency of the highest point of displacement of the acoustic signal measured in Hz. c) Initial Intensity (II) - initial intensity of the acoustic signal recorded by sonar Doppler during the swallowing event, ranging from 10 dB to 140 dB. d) Peak Intensity (PI) - peak of the wave recorded by sonar Doppler during the swallowing event, amplitude of the sound signal, ranging from 10 dB to 140 dB. e) Swallowing Duration (T) - time elapsed from swallow apnea to larynx descent in post-swallow exhalation, completing the full swallowing cycle, from the beginning to the end of the acoustic signal, measured in seconds. [22-26, 33-35] The numbers 1 and 2, representing liquid and nectar consistencies, respectively, were added to the abbreviations of the variables as given above, yielding the following symbols: IF1, PF1, II1, FI1, and T1 for those variables during swallowing of the liquid consistency; IF2, PF2, II2, FI2, and T2 for those variables during swallowing of the nectar consistency.The graphical representation of the five variables (initial and peak frequencies, initial and peak intensities, swallowing time) for both groups studied using the Doppler sonar is presented in Figure 3.

The best audio and video recording sample of each child was selected for analysis of frequency, intensity and duration of the swallowing.The swallowing sounds were captured at the same time as the VFSS was performed so that both could later be analysed synchronously, correlating the swallowing movement to the sound recording. Table 1 correlates this pattern of swallowing sounds with anatomical structural movements as seen in the VFSS, in the manner previously described by Morinière.[36]

Statistical Analysis: The variables are expressed as mean (+standard deviation) and median (range). To estimate the difference between values, both the Student T test and the Wilcoxon test for the nonparametric data were used. A significance level of 5% was used.

Results: The study population was composed of 21 children with cerebral palsy and 21 children without neuro-motor impairment. Classified according to age, 7 (33.3%) were between 2 and 5 years, 6 (28.6%) between 6 and 10 years, and 8 (38.1%) 11 to 15 years. Classified according to type of cerebral palsy, 2 children (9.5%) had hemiplegia and 19 (90.5%) tetraplegia. Classified according to severity of dysphagia, 16 (76.1%) demonstrated mild dysphagia, 2 (9.5%) demonstrated moderate dysphagia, and 3 (14.4%) demonstrated severe dysphagia. Abnormalities in the oral phase were observed in 21 children (100%) during the clinical evaluation, and impairments in pharyngeal phase were observed in 5 (23.9%) during VFSS.Aspiration was detected in 5 (24%) of the children in the study, the liquid consistency being aspirated by 4 children, the nectar consistency being aspirated by 5 children, and the pudding consistency being aspirated by 3 children.Multiple swallows were observed in 20 (95%) of the children that participated in the study.Characteristics of the sound waves generated during swallowing among the groups studied are presented in Table 2.Initial Frequency during liquid swallowing (IF1), was significantly higher in cerebral palsy patients as compared to that of the control group (mean 777.08 ± 98.87 Hzcompared to 706.00 ± 57.44; p=0.02). Initial Frequencyduring nectar consistency swallowing (IF2), was notsignificantly differentbetween the two groups.

Peak Frequency during liquid swallowing (PF1) was significantly lower in cerebral palsy patients as compared to that of the control group (mean 1035.37 ± 70.10 Hz compared to 1095.67 + 22.19; p=0.001). Peak Frequency during nectar swallowing (PF2) was likewise significantly lower in cerebral palsy patients as compared to that of the control group (mean 1039.51 ± 71.47 Hz compared to 1083.62 + 30.46; p=0.003).

Initial Intensity during liquid swallowing (II1) was significantly higher in cerebral palsy patients as compared to that of the control group (mean 66.51 ± 7.60 dB compared to 61.0 +4.53; p=0.002). Initial Intensity during nectar swallowing (II2), however, was not significantly different between both groups.Peak Intensity during liquid swallowing (PI1) was significantly lower in cerebral palsy patients as compared to that of the control group (mean 84.51 ± 12.10 dB compared to 91.76 +1.75; p=0.016). Peak Intensity during nectar swallowing (PI2) was likewise significantly lower in cerebral palsy patients as compared to that of the control group (mean 88.18 ± 3.79 dB compared to 90.81+2.40; p=0.003).

Time elapsed during liquid swallowing (T1) was significantly greater in the group with cerebral palsy as compared to that of the control group (median 1.23s (0.54-2.77) compared to 0.92s (0.53 - 1.43); p=0.007). Time elapsed during nectar swallowing (T2) was significantly greater in cerebral palsy patients compared to that of the control group (median 1.64s (0.76-2.52) compared to 0.89s (0.45 - 1.37); p=0.001).In summary, all variables were significantly different among children with cerebral palsy during liquid swallowing. As for the nectar consistency, all variables except for initial frequency (IF2) and initial intensity (II2)were significantly different between the groups.

Discussion:In order to evaluate the swallowing sounds using sonar Doppler, a case-control study comparing children with cerebral palsy to a paired control group of children without neuromotor impairment was conducted. This study identified and compared the specific characteristics of the sound waves of sonar Doppler captured during VFSS in children with and without cerebral palsy. The average initial frequency (FI1) and initial intensity (FI1)during swallowing, which represent the elevation of the larynx at the beginning of the pharyngeal phase of swallowing, were greater for the group of children with cerebral palsy, a difference in mobility and muscular force being observed during this phase. This suggests the need for greater protection for the upper respiratory tract at the moment of liquidswallowing, with a greater elevation and maintenance of the larynx. This might be suggested in sonar Doppler by the elevation/ higher index of the sound curve at the beginning of the pharyngeal phase. In addition to all the oral irregularities observed in the children during the VFSS, irregularities in the control and mobility of the pharyngeal phase were also observed.

The Sonar Doppler readings for Peak Frequency (PF) and Peak Intensity (PI) represent the opening of the cricopharyngeal muscle (upper oesophageal sphincter). Comparing both the study group and the control for the two consistencies, both of these readings were smaller for the group with cerebral palsy. This may indicate a functioning of the upper oesophageal sphincter which is almost normal, as was observed during the VFSS evaluation.

A comparison of the sonar Doppler waves revealed that swallowing duration (corresponding to the time elapsed from swallow apnea to descent of the larynx) was longer in the cerebral palsy group for both consistencies. These data agree with those reported by other studies in the literature, as should be expected, since children with cerebral palsy demonstrate great difficulty in oral and pharyngeal mobility and thus require a greater amount of time to ingest food.[4,6,8,17-21]

As for the nectar consistency, the initial frequency (IF2) and initial intensity (II2) in cerebral palsy patients were not significantly different when compared to the readings for the control group. These findings suggest that the improvement in the perception of food in the oral cavity given by a thicker consistency may provide improved handling and elevation of the larynx, causing the swallow to be triggered more quickly. Another possible explanation for the improved responses with nectar is the slower flow of the liquid, which children can then handle more competently. The effect of thicker consistencies has been visualised and described during VFSS.[4,6,8,17-21,37,38]

No sound patterns suggesting aspiration were recognised in this study, although results may be limited by the fact that aspiration was detected in only five children in the present study.A fewother studies have been published which analyse swallowing sounds using sonar Doppler.Abdulmassih analysed the variables of frequency, time, and intensity for swallowing sounds as well, comparing the results obtained from two groups of 30 adults, one with and the other without spinocerebellar ataxia.She noticed significant differences in sound signal wave patterns during swallowing, similar to those found in the patients with cerebral palsy in the current study. They also observed a higher Initial Frequency (IF) and Initial Intensity (II), as well as higher Peak Frequency (PF) and Peak Intensity (PI) in their patients with cerebral palsy. The results were attributed to motor dysfunction.[35]

Sória compared the acoustic parameters of swallowing among different ages. She correlated swallowing and aging by analysing 75 elderly adults and 72 healthy young and middle-aged adults, obtaining results regarding muscular movement reduction in the elderly adults that were similar to those of our patients with cerebral palsy. A decrease in speed at the onset of the pharyngeal phase with decreased laryngeal elevation (IF and II) and increased swallowing duration (T) were observed in the elderly adults, just as was observed in the group of cerebral palsy patients in the present study.[33]

Cagliari analysed swallowing sounds of 90 children without oropharyngeal dysfunction between 2 and 15 years of age, describing differences related to age. The frequency and intensity of the sound patterns generated during swallowing were lower in the younger group and increased with age. She believed these differences were probably due to the difference in larynx size. Higher frequency and intensity and shorter swallowing time correspond to a better performance in the swallowing process.[26] The opposite occurred in the cerebral palsy patients in the present study.No further studies with sonar Doppler assessing the paediatric population with dysphagia were found.

A limitation of this study was the use of only 5 ml food with barium. The present study group was composed of children under 15 years of age (50% under 10 years), with a low BMI indexand difficulties handling oral barium.A higher volume would have been too difficult for many of the patients. Nevertheless, the sonar Doppler analysis conducted by Sóri comparing the swallowing sounds of adults using 5 and 10 ml samples of different consistencies found no differences between the data generated by the two different volumes.[33]

These data suggest that the swallowing process in cerebral palsy patients, besides being slower as a result of oropharyngeal dysphagia, also results in great difficulty in the control of muscle tone and the mobility of the muscular structures involved in the process. Additional studies are needed in order to standardise the curves and simultaneously analyse the sound and image of the swallowing process using specific software. A non-invasive, fast, and accessible way of assessing children with cerebral palsy, especially in order to determine risk of prandial aspiration, could substantially improve their quality of life.

Conclusion: The acoustic parameters analysed from the swallowing sound patterns captured by the sonar Doppler from children with cerebral palsy demonstrated statistical significance when compared to the population of children without neuromotor impairment. Swallowing duration is significantly longer for the group of children with cerebral palsy for both liquid and nectar consistencies. Significant differences are observed with the liquid consistency for all variables (time, frequency and intensity) as well as with the nectar consistency for the variables of time and peak frequency. Although significant differences were seen in the sonar Doppler evaluation of children with cerebral palsy, the study was unable to identify a wave pattern which suggests prandial aspiration in this small group of patients. Either a larger group study of patients with cerebral palsy and pharyngeal dysphagia or alternative methods of sound signal analysis are needed in order to address this issue.

References

1. Logeman JA. Swallowing disorders. Best Pract Res Cl Ga. 2007; 21:563-73. doi: 10.1016/j.bpg.2007.03.006

1. Santini CS. Neurogenic dysphagia. In: Furkim AM & Santini CS. Oropharyngeal dysphagia. Pró- Fono. São Paulo; 1999:19-34.

3. Aurelio SR, Genaro KF, Macedo-Filho EDF. Comparative analysis of swallowing patterns in children with cerebral palsy and normal children. Braz J Otorhinolaryngol. 2002; 68:167-73.

4. Furkim AM, Behlau M, Weckx LLM. Clinical and videofluoroscopic evaluation of swallowing in children with cerebral palsy. ArqNeuropsiquiatr. 2003; 61:611-6.

5. Vasconcelos RLM, Moura TL, Campos TF, Lindquist ARR, Guerra RO. Evaluation of the functional performance of children with cerebral palsy according to levels of motor impairment. RevBrasFisioter. 2009; 13:390-7.

6. Viana CIO, Suzuki HS. Cerebral palsy: analysis of swallowing patterns before and after speech therapy intervention. Revista CEFAC. 2011; 13:790-800.

7. Arvedson JC. Feeding children with cerebral palsy and swallowing difficulties.EJCN.2013; 67:9-12. doi:10.1038/ejcn.2013.224.

8. Penny LM, RiskiJE, Glascott J, Johnson V.Videofluoroscopic assessment of dysphagia in children with severe spastic cerebral palsy. Dysphagia. 1994; 9:174-9.

9. Padovani AR, Moraes DP, Mangili LD Andrade CRF. Speech and hearing therapy protocol for assessing risk of dysphagia (PARD) Rev Soc Bras Fonoaudiol. 2007; 12:199-205.

10. Quintella T and Silva AA. In: Furkim AM & Santini CS. Oropharyngeal dysphagia. Pró-Fono. São Paulo, 1999: 61-96.

11. Groher ME. In: Furkim AM & Santini CS. Oropharyngeal dysphagia. Pró-Fono. São Paulo, 1999: 97-107.

12. Gonçalves MIR and Vidigal MLN. In: Furkim AM & Santini CS. Oropharyngeal dysphagia. Pró- Fono. São Paulo, 1999: 189-201.

13. Furkim AM, Duarte ST, Sacca AFB, Sória FS. The use of cervical auscultation in inferring tracheal aspiration in children with cerebral palsy. Rev CEFAC. 2009; 11:624-9.

14. Eicher PPS, Mano CJ, Fox CA, Kerwin ME.Impact of cervical auscultation on accuracy of clinical evaluation in predicting penetration/aspiration in paediatric population.Minute-second workshop on cervical auscultation. Mc Lean, Virginia. 1994:28-32.

15. Mckaig TN. Cervical and thoracic auscultation. In: Furkim AM & Santini CS. Oropharyngeal dysphagia. Pró-Fono. São Paulo, 1999:171-87.

16. Manrique D, Melo ECM, Buhler RB. Nasofibrolaryngoscopic changes in swallowing in chronic non-progressive encephalopathy. J Pediat. 2002; 78:67-70.

17. Marrara JL, Duca AP, Dantas RO, Trawitzki LVV. Lima RAC, Pereira JC. Swallowing in children with neurological disorders: clinical and videofluoroscopic evaluation. Pró-Fono.2008; 20:231-6.

18. Su CL, Chen SL, Tsai SW, Tseng FE, Chang SC, Huang YH, Lin YH. Efficacy of predicting videofluoroscopic results in dysphgic patients with severe cerebral palsy using de Mann assesment of swallowing ability. Am J Phys Med Rehabil.2016; 95:270-6.

19. Engel-Koek L, Erasmus CE, Hulst KCM, ArvedsonJc, Groot IJM, Swart BJM (2014) Children with central and peripheral neurologic disorders have distinguishable patterns of dysphagia onvideofluoroscopic swallow study. Journal of Child Neurology.2014; 29:646-53.doi: 10.1177/0883073813501871.

20. Wright RER, Wright FR, Carson CA. Videofluoroscopic assessment in children with severe cerebral palsy presenting with dysphagia.PediatrRadiot.1996; 26:720-2.

21. Kim JS, Ham ZA, Song DH, Oh HM. Characteristics of dysphagia in children with cerebral palsy related to Gross Motor Function. Am J Phys Med Rehabil.2013; 92: 912-9.

22. Hamlet SL, Nelson RJ, Patterson RL.Interpreting the sounds of swallowing; fluid flow through the cricopharyngeus. Ann OtolRhinolLaryngol. 1990; 99:749-52.

23. Hamlet SL, Patterson RL, Fleming SM, Jones LA.Sounds of Swallowing following total laryngectomy.Dysphagia.1992; 7:160-5.

24. Cichero JAY, Murdoch BE. The physiologic cause of swallowing sounds: answers from heart sounds and vocal tract acoustics. Dysphagia.1998; 13:39-52.

25. Santos RS, Macedo-Filho ED. Sonar Doppler as an instrument of deglutition evaluation. Intl Arch Otorhinolaryngology.2006; 10:182-91.

26. Cagliari CF; Jurkiewicz AL; Santos RS; Marques JM. Doppler sonar analysis of swallowing sounds in normal paediatric individuals. Braz J Otorhinolaryngol. 2009; 75:706-15.

27. Behlau & Michalis. VoxMetria - Software for Analysing Voice and Vocal Quality. CTS Informática. 2003.

28. ASHA. Guidelines for Speech-Language Pathologists Performing Videofluoroscopic Swallowing Studies.ASHA Special Interest Division 13, Swallowing and Swallowing Disorders. Dikeman K, Green J, HISS S, Inman A, Kelchner L, Lazarus C, Miller C.Dysphagia.2004. doi:10.1044/policy.GL2004-00050.

29. ADA. National Dysphagia Diet: Standardisation for Optimal Care. American Dietetic Association. 2002.

30. Ott DJ, Hodge RG, Pikna LA, Chen MY, Gelfand DW. Modified barium swallow: clinical and radiographic correlation and relation to feeding recommendations. Dysphagia.1996; 11:187-90.

31. Takahashi K, Groher ME, Michi K. Methodology for detecting swallowing sounds. Dysphagia.1994; 9:54-62.

32. Youmans SR, Stierwalt JAG. An acoustic profile of normal swallowing.Dysphagia.2005; 20:195-209.

33. Sória FS, Silva RG, Furkim AM. Acoustic analysis of oropharyngeal swallowing using doppler sonar. Braz J Otorhinolaryngol. 2016; 82:39-46.

34. Lagos HNC, Santos RS, Abdulmassih EMS, Gallinea LF, Langone M. Characterisation of swallowing sounds with the use of sonar Doppler in full-term and preterm newborns. Intl Arch Otorhinolaryngology.2013; 17:383-6.doi: 10.1055/s-0033-1353369.

35. Abdulmassih EMS, Teive HAG, Santos RS. The evaluation of swallowing in patients with spinocerebellar ataxia and oropharyngeal dysphagia: A comparison study of videofluoroscopy and sonar Doppler. Intl Arch Otorhinolaryngol.2013; 17:66-73.doi: 10.7162/S1809-97772013000100012.

36. Morinière S, Boiron M, Alison D, Makris P, Beutter P. Origin of the sound components during pharyngeal swallowing in normal subjects. Dysphagia. 2008; 23: 267-73. doi: 10.1007/s00455- 007-9134-z.

37. Lustre NS, Freira TRB, Silverio CC. Oral transit time measurements in children with cerebral palsy of different motor levels and their relationship with the degree of severity for dysphagia. ACR. 2013; 18:155-61.

38. Vivone GP, Tavares MMM, Bartolomeu RS, Nemr K, Chiappetta ALML. Analysis of food consistency and swallowing time in children with spastic quadriplegic cerebral palsy. Rev CEFAC. 2007; 4:504-11.

Table 1

TABLE 1 -CORRELATION OF SWALLOWING SOUND PATTERNSSTO ANATOMICAL STRUCTURAL MOVEMENT SEEN IN VFS

SWALLOWINGSOUND PATTERNS(DOPPLER)	ANATOMIC STRUCTURES (VFS)
Initial Frequency (IF) and Initial Intensity (II)	Elevation of the larynx, beginning of the pharyngeal phase of swallowing
Peak Frequency (PF) and Peak Intensity (PI)	Opening of the cricopharyngeal muscle (upper oesophageal sphincter)
Time (T) - elapsed time from beginning to end of the acoustic signal	Structures return to original position (descent of the larynx)

Table 2

TABLE 2 - CHARACTERISTICS OF THE SWALLOWING SOUND WAVES OBSERVED BY SONAR DOPPLER

CONSISTENCY AND VARIABLE	STUDY GROUP (n = 21)	CONTROL GROUP (n = 21)	P
Liquid			
Initial Frequency 1 (IF1) Hz	777.08 + 98.87	706.00 + 57.44	0.002[*]
Peak Frequency 1 (PF1) Hz	1035.37 + 70.10	1095.67 + 22.19	0.001[*]
Initial Intensity 1 (II1) dB	66.51 + 7.60	61.00 + 4.53	0.002[*]
Peak Intensity 1 (PI1) dB	84.51 + 12.10	91.76 + 1.75	0.016[*]
Time1 (T1) s	1.23 (0.54 -2.77)	0.92 (0.53 -1.43)	0.007[**]
Nectar	759.77 + 135.93	719.74 + 59.81	0

Initial Frequency 2 (IF2) Hz			.063*
Peak Frequency 2 (PF2) Hz	1039.51 + 71.47	1083.62 + 30.46	0
			.003*
Initial Intensity 2 (II2) dB	66.33 + 8.76	62.08 + 4.72	0
			.06*
Peak Intensity 2 (PI2) dB	88.18 + 3.79	90.81 + 2.40	0
			.003*
Time 2 (T2) s	1.64 (0.76 -2.52)	0.89 (0.45 - 1.37)	0
			.001

Note: [a] Dependent Student Test, [aa] Test of Wilcoxon, $p < 0.05$ was considered significant

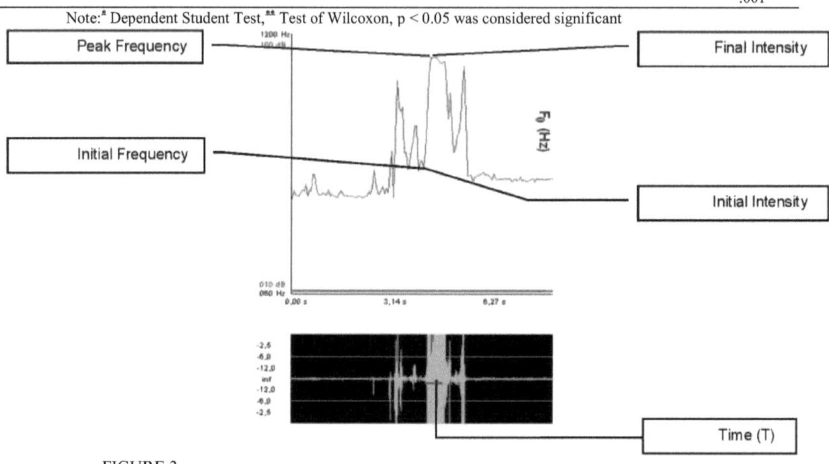

FIGURE 3

Figure 3 - Graphical representation of swallowing sound variables captured by the Doppler sonar

Note: s = seconds; Hz = Hertz; db = decibel; FO = frequency; PF = peak frequency; IF = initial frequency; II = initial intensity; FI = final intensity; T = time

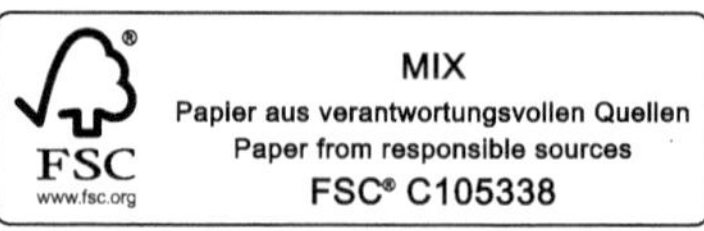

Printed by Books on Demand GmbH, Norderstedt / Germany